AN INTRODUCTION TO THE
Management of Information Standards *for* Health Care Organizations

JOINT COMMISSION

RA
971.6
.I585
1995

ACU 8652

Joint Commission Mission

The mission of the Joint Commission on Accreditation of Healthcare Organizations is to improve the quality of care provided to the public.

© 1995 by the Joint Commission on Accreditation of Healthcare Organizations

All rights reserved. No part of this book may be reproduced in any form or by any means without written permission from the publisher.

Printed in the U.S.A.   5 4 3 2 1

Requests for permission to reprint or make copies of any part of this book should be addressed to:
Permissions Editor
Joint Commission on Accreditation of Healthcare Organizations
One Renaissance Blvd.
Oakbrook Terrace, IL 60181

ISBN: 0-86688-429-7

Library of Congress Catalog Card Number: 94-73293

Contents

	Introduction 1
Chapter 1.	An Overview of the Standards 7
Chapter 2.	A Detailed Look at the Standards 23
Chapter 3.	An Overview of the Survey Process 123
Appendix A.	The "Management of Information" Chapter from the 1995 *CAMH* 163
Appendix B.	An Overview of the Joint Commission's Indicator Measurement System 283
Appendix C.	Additional Resources 289
Appendix D.	Management of Information Terms 307
Appendix E.	Sample Information Management Plan 311
	Index 327

Introduction

When a 55-year-old man is discharged from a health care network after a successful bypass procedure, he might commend the skills of his surgeon and the attentiveness of his nurse. Six months later, he might ascribe his new-found energy to a nutritionist who helped him change his eating habits.

As this example illustrates, patients generally associate good health outcomes with provider expertise. Rarely do patients connect their outcomes to the effective capture of data or information or methods for linking different data sets. However, the management of information is as crucial to the outcome of any procedure as physician skill and medical equipment.

For example, the surgeon in the case above recorded and relied on data in the patient record, such as vital signs and family history, to make an accurate assessment and determine treatment. The nutritionist consulted with the patient's surgeon and nurses to determine a proper nutrition plan. She then obtained appropriate materials from the resource center to use in educating the patient about his diet.

In addition, the health care network that provided the patient's care belongs to an external database. Organization leaders had been using information from this database to continuously compare their cardiac outcomes with those of similar institutions. As a result, the organizations were able to identify opportunities for improving outcomes and lowering costs of bypass procedures. The leaders assigned a team with representatives from across the network (clinics, hospitals, and home care providers) to develop a critical path for bypass procedures that followed the patient through the continuum of care. The team began by studying the clinical literature and was able to adapt several "best practices" that helped decrease length of stay. Meanwhile, after reviewing aggregate data, the pharmacy was able to recommend several medications that were less expensive but just as effective for bypass patients.

In this example, we see that data and information are crucial resources at every step of a procedure. Without patient-based information, caregivers would have had difficulty making the correct assessment or administering the proper treatment. And, without comparative data and information such as that provided by the external database, leaders may not have identified opportunities for improvement in their bypass procedures. The case, therefore, illustrates the intrinsic link between the coordination and use of information and the important functions a health care organization carries out—from patient assessment to patient education, and from performance improvement to the management of human resources.

The prominent role of information in health care organizations, as shown in our example, has greatly increased in recent years as has the expectation that these organizations would manage and link different types of information systematically. These expectations are voiced by purchasers and patients who demand information regarding costs and outcomes. To meet these demands, organizations are capturing and transmitting data about various aspects of their performance. Additionally, as communities across the country move toward managed and/or integrated care, health care organizations are contemplating how to design information processes that cross the care continuum.

These demands and needs, representative of the issues that have arisen in the evolving health care climate, have led many hospitals and other health care organizations to respond by fundamentally rethinking the way they do business. For example, some hospitals are re-engineering traditional nursing units into patient care centers, where all services (nursing, laboratory, and so forth) are brought as close to the patient as possible. Organizational changes, such as this one, also call for the process changes related to the management of information. Also, the growth in information technology is encouraging many organizations to reexamine the way their patient information is managed. This new technology (for example, computerized patient records, local area networks) is helping to make visions from the past a real possibility in the near future (for example, community health information networks). It is important to note, however, that with the promise of this possible future come many demands.

To meet these future demands, health care organizations can use the new Joint Commission management of information standards as a framework for designing information processes. The objectives of the standards will mirror the objectives of health care organizations as they examine their current information processes. These include:

- More timely and easier access to complete information throughout the organization;
- Improved data accuracy;
- Demonstrated balance of proper levels of security versus ease of access;
- Use of compiled data, along with external knowledge bases and comparative data, to pursue opportunities for improvement and identify current best practices;
- Redesign of important information-related processes to improve efficiency; and
- Greater collaboration and information-sharing to enhance patient care.

The new standards help leaders and staff envision the management of information as an organizationwide function focused on anticipating and meeting the organization's information needs.

■ Chapter Organization

This publication provides an overview of the Joint Commission's new management of information standards. The first two chapters describe the requirements in detail. The third chapter gives an overview of how these standards will be surveyed. Because these standards are being phased in (refer to current scoring guidelines for details), this book is designed to help organizations understand what would be a reasonable expectation for compliance in 1995 and 1996 and what will be required in the next five years. In addition, the appendices to this book include a sample information management plan, a list of other resources, and an overview of the Joint Commission's Indicator Measurement System (IMSystem).

This book is primarily directed to information management directors and medical records professionals within hospitals and health care networks. However, the scope of the management of information function makes this publication of interest to many other staff members, including organization leaders, quality improvement directors, medical librarians, risk managers, utilization management directors, chief financial officers, and human resource directors. In addition, since the management of information standards are similar across all Joint Commission accreditation manuals, other types of health care organizations (for example, home care, mental health, ambulatory, and long term care) should find this publication of value.

This book is one of many educational resources the Joint Commission plans on providing the field in regard to the management of information standards. We hope that this publication will answer your questions and address your concerns about the new requirements. However, if you have a particular question that is not answered in this book, please contact the Joint Commission's Department of Interpretation at 708/916-5900. Joint Commission staff members will be happy to help you. In addition, if you have any ideas or feedback regarding future publications related to the management of information, please contact the Department of Publications at 708/916-5438.

CHAPTER 1

An Overview of the Standards

The management of information standards essentially ask the following three questions:
- Are your internal and external users getting the *correct information*?
- Are they receiving this information in an *effective, efficient, and accurate manner*?
- Are they receiving this information at the *right time*?

The Joint Commission's ultimate concern in these standards is the performance of management of information processes. Before an organization can respond to these questions, it needs to consider the issues addressed in the "Management of Information" chapter of the 1995 *Accreditation Manual for Hospitals (AMH)*. To understand those issues, it is helpful to track the development of the management of information standards.

■ How the Standards Were Developed

In 1986, the Joint Commission began to redesign its accreditation system. For years, accredited organizations had been complaining that surveys were too retrospective and too focused on documentation. During the reevaluation, Joint Commission staff and board members worked to determine the proper focus for measurement in an accreditation system. They found that an accreditation system, in which the focal point is *performance*, would reflect the growing emphasis on results (that is, outcomes) in the health care industry. *These results indicate the quality of care an organization provides.*

Since the turn of the century, organizations have been using standards compliance as a basic measure of health care quality. Though this is one method for predicting the likelihood of future compliance (that is, an organization's *capacity* for performance), it does not provide the information that purchasers and patients request about an organization's *actual* performance. With the cost of health care rapidly increasing, purchasers and patients want to know *what* they are buying and its value. They also want to know if an organization is providing the right care in an efficient manner.

To assess an organization's actual performance, it is necessary to measure how well an organization carries out the vital activities and important functions involved in the delivery of care. To identify these activities, Joint Commission staff members consulted with health care experts from across the country. After these discussions, a new functional framework for the standards emerged. This framework recognizes that health care organizations are integrated systems, not a collection of independent departments and services. Previously, the Joint Commission accreditation manuals were designed around the major departments and services within a health care organization. The new functional structure encourages interdepartmental collaboration for delivering quality patient care.

As the standards reevaluation progressed, two sets of important functions were identified—those directly experienced by patients and those carried on behind the scenes. The first part of the 1995 *AMH*, "Patient-Focused Functions," traces the patient's pathway through a continuum of care. These standards focus on the functions and processes directly related to patient care. The second part of the *AMH*, "Organizational Functions," identifies those functions and processes that, although not directly experienced by patients, are vital to the organization's ability to provide high-quality patient care. In addition, the third section of the *AMH*, "Structures with Functions," addresses four organizational structures necessary to a health care organization: Governing Body, Administration, Medical Staff, and Nursing.

Because a health care organization depends on information to carry out its patient care and other activities, the management of information was identified as one of the most vital organizational functions. This importance led the Joint Commission to implement a standards development process for management of information standards. To help develop standards that measure how effectively and efficiently an organization managed this important resource, the Joint Commission assembled a task force of experts in the management of information from across the country, including information management specialists, data processing specialists, and data and information users. The task force worked with staff to research and develop a broad, visionary set of principles that sets forth clear goals for the management of information for all health care organizations. Standards were then proposed based on these principles.

These standards went through several extensive internal and external review cycles, including review by members of health care organizations, national professional organizations, government agencies, and other concerned parties. Many changes were suggested and adopted. The last step was approval by the Joint Commission's Board of Commissioners, which is composed of seven public members and professionals from member organizations—the American Hospital Association, American Medical Association, American College of Physicians, American College of Surgeons, and American Dental Association.

The "Management of Information" chapter first appeared in the 1994 *Accreditation Manual for Hospitals*. Similar chapters appear in the 1995 standards manuals for health care networks, home care organizations, and mental health organizations. In 1996, the chapter will appear in the ambulatory health care and long term care manuals. The requirements are very similar across all manuals, although some language and scoring changes have been made to reflect differences among these settings, populations served, and organizational structures.

■ The Standards as a Planning Guide

The management of information standards recognize the prominent role that the management of information plays in an organization's ability to function. Without the effective and efficient management of information, organizations cannot properly deliver patient care or carry out other important activities, such as performance improvement. Thus, the Joint Commission views the management of information as not only helping organizations to meet external demands, but also the critical demands arising in any organization's internal environment. Therefore, organizational leaders should view this function as an activity that needs to be planned for, just like human, material, and financial resources management.

■ Meeting Expectations

To help guide organizational leaders through this planning, the standards focus on key processes for meeting internal and external information needs. Within the next several years, the Joint Commission expects organizations to ensure that their management of information processes:

- *Are based on the organization's vision, mission, and strategic plan.* Because the management of information is so closely intertwined with the accomplishment of an organization's mission and vision, it is crucial that any informational needs planning be integrated with the organization's strategic plans.

- *Respond to the needs of different users of information.* The ultimate judges of how well these processes perform are the users. This includes staff, patients, providers, external regulators, and others who may have various needs related to the capture, analysis, interpretation, transformation, and transmission of information.
- *Provide the different types of information required by users.* Organizations need to assess the different types of information they manage, including patient-specific, aggregate, knowledge-based, and comparative.
- *Ensure that the necessary processes are in place to provide the different types of information.* The effective management of information requires that organizations have the following processes in place for each type of information:
  - identification of data sources;
  - capture of data;
  - analysis of data;
  - interpretation of data;
  - transformation of data into information; and
  - transmission of data.
- *Provide for the different uses of information.* Staff members use different types of information in various ways, including clinical decision making, patient education, organizational decision making, research, and performance improvement.

Essentially, these expectations of an organization's management of information processes trace the flowchart of the management of information function (see Figure 1, page 12). The Joint Commission expects organizations to have processes established that reflect the activities identified in this flowchart.

An Organizationwide Scope

Previously in this book, management of information was identified as a prominent organizational function that crosses interdepartmental lines. As with all of the new function-focused

FIGURE 1 Management of Information Function

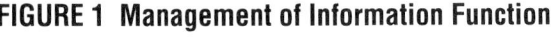

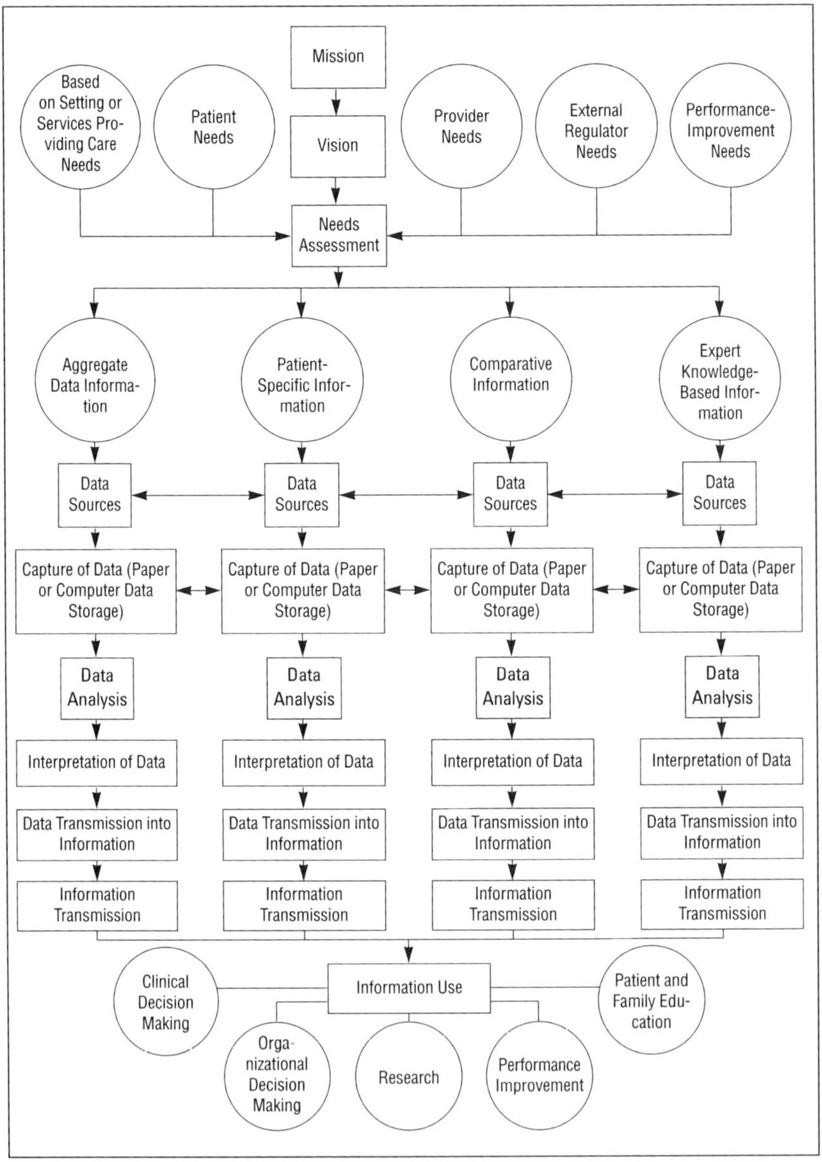

This flowchart graphically represents most of the important activities and processes, particularly the risk points, in the management of information function.

standards, the Joint Commission is asking your organization to rethink the way you view and manage services. In this case, that would be the way you view and manage information.

To illustrate this shift in perspective, we can look for an example to the former "Medical Records" chapter in the program manuals that dealt with patient-based information, and the former "Professional Library Services" chapter that dealt with knowledge-based information. By organizing and segregating these standards according to departments, we may have encouraged organizations to manage different types of information separately—to create data dynasties.

The new "Management of Information" chapter addresses this concern by encouraging an integrated approach to the management of information. Just as the "Assessment of Patients" chapter in the manuals encourages different disciplines to interact when assessing a patient's care needs, the "Management of Information" chapter stimulates organizations to manage different types of data and information simultaneously.

The implications of viewing information as an organization-wide resource are significant. As staff members begin to understand that the principles articulated in the first six standards of the "Management of Information" chapter apply to managing all types of information, they can learn to combine their efforts. As a result, some organizations can decentralize their information services processes or create mechanisms for staff members to more actively participate in the design and improvement of processes related to the management of information.

Processes Versus Technology

The new standards focus on the processes organizations need to have in place to effectively manage information. A process is a series of interrelated activities or steps that lead to a desired outcome. However, due to the nonprescriptive nature of the standards, they do not focus on the technology used in these processes. For example, staff members follow a series of steps to move data from one area of the organization to another. In many instances, the use of information technology might facilitate this process. For example, a health care network might have local area networks (LANs) in place to facilitate data transmission among its different entities. However, it important to note that technology is simply a tool that staff members use to get from step A to step B.

As the new standards are not prescriptive of the types of technology used in an organization's management of information processes, staff can also use various other tools to help them carry out processes, including data collection forms, critical pathways, and the like. In addition, computers may also play a prominent role in an organization's information processes as many organizations are now using some type of computer support. However, these standards are as equally applicable in heavily computerized organizations as they are in organizations with no computer support.

The standards have wide applicability across diverse environments because they are based on underlying principles of the management of information. For example, standard IM.6 requires organizations to establish linkages among data sets. This linkage reflects a basic concept of the management of information—that is, do not create or maintain isolated data sets that can't be woven together. Many organizations assume that this requirement means establishing electronic linkages. They can, however, construct manual linkages to fulfill this management of information principle. This example illustrates the paramount importance of an organization's processes.

This basic concept of developing and performing sound processes is at the heart of all Joint Commission standards. That is, even though the quality- and cost-conscious health care environment demands efficient processes and though technology's usefulness cannot be denied, leaders should not become so enamored of technology that they forget about the underlying processes. As Thomas H. Davenport, Partner and Director of

Research at the Ernst & Young Center for Information Technology and Strategy in Boston, has warned: "Information technology has a polarizing effect...bedazzled [information technology] departments frequently become prisoners of their own fascination, constructing elaborate technology architectures and enterprise information models to guide systems development.... But such technocratic solutions often specify the minutiae of machinery while disregarding how people in organizations go about acquiring, sharing, and making use of information."[1]

Again, it must be stressed that the Joint Commission is more interested in the processes your organization uses to acquire, share, and make use of information than in the technology used to perform the processes. That is, technology is considered to be just one component in meeting the intent of the standards. To manage information and strive to comply with the standards, organizations will use a certain tool to help implement its processes. This might be a paper and pencil, or it might be a computer. However, more important than the tool used are the underlying processes an organization sets up to manage information effectively. For example, what steps does your organization take when capturing data? How do you establish data needs and definitions? How do you test data for reliability, and information for validity? These types of questions help illustrate the concept that effective management of information occurs mainly because staff members design good processes.

An Emphasis on Performance

The emphasis on the integrity of underlying processes and their support of the management of information is mirrored by the emphasis on performance in the standards. The Joint Commission will be able to measure the effectiveness of an organization's processes by assessing the organization's compliance with the new standards. In measuring performance, the surveyors assess standards compliance in a variety of ways, including interviews, observations, and documentation review. They use a five-point scale to indicate an organization's level of compliance with a standard. Each score, 1 through 5, corresponds to a defined level of compliance:

SCORE 1 **Substantial compliance** indicates that the organization consistently meets *all* major provisions of the standard (some provisions may be in the intent).

SCORE 2 **Significant compliance** indicates that the organization meets *most* provisions of the standard.

SCORE 3 **Partial compliance** indicates that the organization meets *some* provisions of the standard.

SCORE 4 **Minimal compliance** indicates that the organization meets *few* provisions of the standard.

SCORE 5 **Noncompliance** indicates that the organization *fails to meet* the provisions of the standard.

NA **Not applicable** indicates that the standard does not apply to the organization.

The Joint Commission's new emphasis on performance is supported by the flexibility and nonprescriptiveness of the standards. The flexibility can be clearly seen in the scoring guidelines (see Appendix A, page 163), which contain a range of compliance and performance-improvement information and offer strategies for fulfilling a standard. These scoring guidelines may also describe options for meeting the intent of a standard that consider differences in the missions, patient populations, and structures of organizations.

This flexibility was incorporated into the standards during the Joint Commission standards revision process. The aim of the revision process was to improve patient care outcomes; therefore, less emphasis is placed on *how* to achieve the objectives of a given standard. Instead, the standards establish a set of consistent performance expectations that an organization is challenged to achieve creatively and consistently. Furthermore, the standards are designed to encourage innovation and provide flexibility; an organization is free to develop strategies and approaches for the management of information that best meet its unique needs and available resources.

The scoring of the standards emphasizes this focus on organizational performance. Lower scores will be given where evidence of performance and/or consistency of performance is lacking. For example, if an organization demonstrates good performance in a given area but that performance is not consistently evident across the organization, they might receive a score of 2 or 3. This indicates the need to address this issue in the future and/or provide a written progress report to the Joint Commission. On the other hand, if an organization has poor performance even when adequate policies and procedures are in place, a score of 4 or 5 may be given. This example shows that actual performance of care will be the focal point for the new standards.

■ What Is Expected in the Next Few Years?

Many standards in the "Management of Information" chapter reflect new standards requirements. The Joint Commission realizes that health care organizations are in varying stages of implementing these requirements. For this reason, many of the more visionary standards are "capped" at a score of 2. This will limit the effect that those scores will have on an organization's accreditation decision. A "cap" defines the maximum impact that the score of a standard can have. For example, in 1995, IM.6.2 is capped at a Score of 2:

IM.6.2

A 1 2 3 4 5 NA   There are internal linkages among information-management processes related to the important patient care and the organizational functions described in this *Manual*.

Although surveyors might assign a score of 3, 4, or 5 to this standard, the impact of the standard on your organization's accreditation decision will be limited to a score of 2. Your organization's accreditation report will, however, provide a supplemental recommendation appropriate for the score assigned by the surveyor. (See Appendix A for a complete explanation of capping and the identification of any specific caps in the management of information standards.)

Organizations have several years to fully comply with those standards considered visionary. Nevertheless, you should begin to address the performance issues these standards raise now. The Joint Commission recognizes that full compliance with these standards will take some time. If the planning and implementation process does not begin immediately, an organization is unlikely to have made sufficient progress by the time subsequent surveys are conducted.

Organizations will receive supplementary recommendations regarding these standards when the intent of the standard is not met. These recommendations are designed to help you improve your organization's performance in the area addressed.

It is up to the particular organization to determine how it will get from its present state to future requirements. Table 1, page 19, provides one possible phased approach for meeting the standards.

■ Framework for Improving Performance

Organizations can use the Joint Commission's framework for improving performance as a guide for approaching the management of information standards.* This framework is the basis of the "Improving Organizational Performance" chapter of the *AMH*.

---

* This book provides only an overview of the Joint Commission's framework for improving performance. Readers interested in learning more about the concepts and methods discussed herein can obtain the recent Joint Commission publication *Framework for Improving Performance: From Principles to Practice*. Copies can be purchased by calling the Joint Commission at 708/916-5800.

TABLE 1 Example Timeline for Complying with the Management of Information Standards

Phase I
- Plan an approach for assessing your organization's information needs.
- Ensure that the organization is in compliance with all "former" standards (for example, IM.7) and/or those not capped.
- Complete needs assessment, including assessment of all those issues identified under IM.1. Identify priorities, including which processes are in place and which processes need to be designed or redesigned.
- Extend participation in external databases.

Phase II
- Based on the plan, improve current management of information processes or design new processes. Implement the plan on a test basis and monitor it to see if it is working well.

Phase III
- Continue monitoring and improving current processes and designing new processes based on the plan.
- Improve support for management of information necessary to improve all the important functions of the organization.

It synthesizes a range of concepts and methods concerning organizational performance that have developed over the last several decades. As illustrated in Figure 2, page 20, this framework incorporates three basic concepts:

- *External environment.* Organizations striving to excel are continuously assessing their environment, eliciting feedback from customers and others, and acting accordingly. The external environment is considered to be the combination of factors outside a health care organization that affect the way an organization designs and carries out its services. For example, when designing processes to manage information, an organization must consider information needs related to health care reform, purchaser or payer requirements, community expectations, and so forth.
- *Internal environment.* "Internal environment" is a blanket term for the functions inside an organization that most greatly

FIGURE 2 Framework for Improving Performance

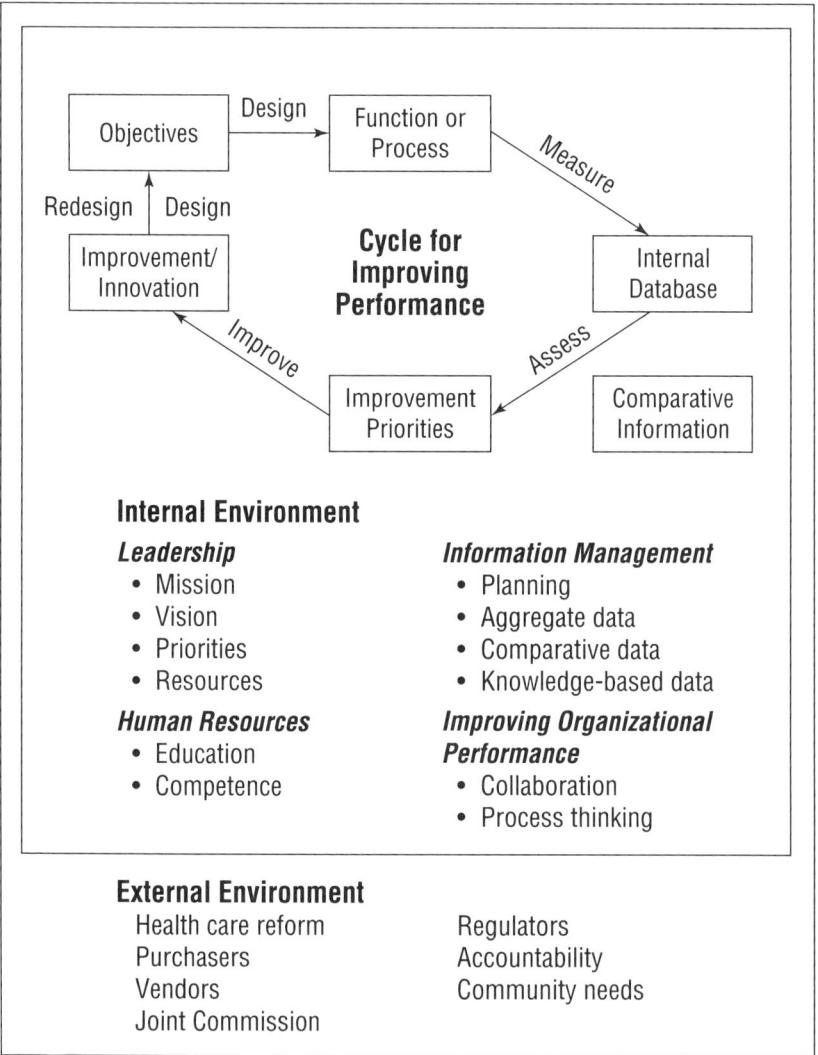

The Joint Commission's framework for improving performance emphasizes the use of external and internal information in the design, measurement, assessment, and improvement of functions.

influence performance. In the *AMH*, four functions are identified within the internal environment: Leadership, Management of Human Resources, Management of Information, and Improvement of Organizational Performance.
- *Cycle for improving performance.* To improve processes and outcomes over time, health care organizations must systematically and scientifically design, measure, assess, and improve their performance. The cycle describes a systematic approach for continuous improvement based on the scientific method.

These three concepts continuously overlap. As an organization moves around the cycle for improving performance, internal and external concerns must be continually taken into account. For example, in setting objectives, an organization might use comparative information, such as that found in an external reference database. It is important to note that once an organization has completed this cycle for a given function or process, the cycle begins again. That is, the objectives are reviewed and perhaps changed. Also, measurement will continue to determine whether improvement has occurred and is sustained.

The building blocks of the improvement cycle are illustrated in Figure 2. Organizations begin by setting *objectives* that define a clear goal or purpose. Based on these objectives, staff members *design* functions or processes. Then, staff members *measure* performance of these processes; an *internal database* can be used to collect performance data over time. Next, staff members *assess* these measurements to identify and prioritize *opportunities for improvement*. One of the tools used to assess performance is *comparative information* from other sources, such as reference databases and practice guidelines. Based on these priorities, staff members create, test, and implement specific *improvements* and innovations, which involve *redesign* or a new *design* of a process.

The cycle for improving performance is flexible and may be applied at a very general level (for example, improving a health care organization) or a very specific level (for example, improving the process for disseminating reports on adverse drug reactions). Thus, the term "function" in Figure 2 can refer to the entire health care organization as a complex system, or it might refer to a multidisciplinary activity such as the management of information. "Process" can refer to a large process, such as the capture of all data and information, or it can apply more specifically to the capture of admissions data. The application of the cycle depends on the improvement project at hand.

Conclusion

One of the first steps organizations might take in complying with the management of information standards is to develop an understanding of information as a resource to be managed. That is, organizations should focus on viewing the management of information as a function—a series of processes—focused on meeting the organization's information needs. The next section examines each set of standards in detail, and answers common questions about the standards.

Reference

1. Davenport TH: Saving IT's Soul: Human-centered information Management. Harv Bus Rev: 119, Mar–Apr 1994.

CHAPTER 2

A Detailed Look at the Standards

In this chapter, management of information standards are grouped into logical sets. For each set, an overview of requirements is provided. This is followed by a brief explanation of the survey process for those standards, and a question-and-answer section. Readers unfamiliar with the survey process might first want to refer to Chapter 3, which gives a step-by-step explanation of the process. In addition, application examples are inserted throughout the chapter. These examples provide practical approaches to complying with the standards.

Planning for the Management of Information (IM.1–IM.1.1.2)

RELATED STANDARDS

IM.1 (Capped at Score 2)

A 1 2 3 4 5 NA Information-management processes are planned and designed to meet the health care organization's internal and external information needs.

IM.1.1 (Capped at Score 2)

A 1 2 3 4 5 NA   The information-management processes within and among organization departments, the medical staff, the administration, and the governing body and with outside services and agencies are appropriate for the organization's size and complexity.

IM.1.1.1 (Capped at Score 2)

A 1 2 3 4 5 NA   Direction, staffing, and material resource allocations are based on the organization's scope and complexity of services provided.

IM.1.1.2 (Capped at Score 2)

A 1 2 3 4 5 NA   Based on the organization's information needs, appropriate staff participate in assessing, selecting, and integrating health care information technology and, as appropriate, using efficient interactive information-management systems for clinical and organizational information.

AN OVERVIEW OF REQUIREMENTS

As stressed in Chapter 1, the Joint Commission expects that an organization's management of information processes will meet the needs of its internal and external users. Obviously, a small, acute care hospital will have different information needs than a health care network that encompasses a hospital, three outpatient clinics, and a home health agency. Therefore, each organization needs to thoroughly assess its needs for the management of information based on its mission, goals, services, personnel, mode(s) of service delivery (for example, hospital, home care, ambulatory), resources, and access to affordable technology.

This analysis should consider the different types of information, along with the different users and uses of that information, that exist throughout the organization. When appropriate, staff members' input should be sought. For example, staff members might be asked if they are receiving the data and information they need to carry out patient care, performance improvement efforts, and other activities.

IM.1 needs to be considered in light of the entire "Management of Information" chapter. This standard simply requires that an organization plan for information needs. The rest of the standards present the essential issues that need to be considered when planning and designing management of information processes. Standards IM.1 through IM.6 describe some basic principles of the management of information that need to be considered (for example, uniform data definitions, data linkages). IM.7 through IM.10 focus on the different types of information that need to be managed (that is, patient-specific, aggregate, knowledge-based, and comparative).

■ How Are These Standards Surveyed?

Surveyors will begin by reviewing any documents (for example, minutes, reports, plans) that describe the needs assessment your organization has carried out or is carrying out, as well as any plans to meet identified needs. During the management of information interview, the surveyor will continue to explore the planning your organization conducted and the resources available to carry out your management of information plans. The surveyor will ask representatives to describe the processes for making information available to those who need it. More details about your organization's planning will be obtained during the Leadership and CEO/Strategic Planning and Resource Allocation interviews.

All of these standards are capped at a score of 2 in 1995. Thus, your organization has a few years to reach full compliance with these standards. An Application Example, on page 31, provides some tips for performing a needs assessment.

COMMON QUESTIONS

Q. What should be considered when assessing management of information processes?
A. The scoring guideline for IM.1 provides a list of issues that should be considered when planning for the management of information (see Table 2, page 27). It covers the different users and uses of information, processes that need to be developed, technology needs, and so forth. Though this list is not exhaustive, it is intended to increase understanding of the standards and illustrate the scope and depth of the management of information function.

Organizations might use this list as a starting point in planning activities to facilitate discussion about assessment needs. You should also consider the issues raised in IM.2 through IM.6. Staff might then develop a plan for assessing management of information needs that is specific to your organization and reflects your mission, vision, and structure.

Q. What time frame should the planning cover?
A. The standards do not require that management of information plans cover any particular time frame. Organizations generally project three to five years into the future.

Q. Do organizations need a separate management of information plan?
A. Not necessarily. If you read the standards carefully, there is no requirement for a written plan entitled "The Information Management Plan." Rather, the standards require a planned approach to the management of information. One way to provide evidence of this planning is to develop a separate plan that describes the processes you have in place (or plan to put in place) for managing different types of information. But the planning might also be reflected in the organization's strategic plan, departmental planning documents, or meeting minutes.

TABLE 2 Checklist for Plan

A management of information needs assessment considers, as appropriate:
Check all that apply.

____ The organization's type, structure, size, and complexity

____ The individuals or groups whom the function is serving or will serve (for example, governance, managers, clinical staff, inpatients and ambulatory patients, patients' families, payers and purchasers, regulatory bodies, accreditation bodies)

____ The support needed for planning purposes

____ The support needed for education services and any research activity

____ Any national and state guidelines for data set parity and connectivity in interfacing information systems

____ The requirements for internal and external transmission of data and information

____ Longitudinal data and information reporting needs

____ The requirements for internally and externally generated data and information to support continuous performance improvement

____ The requirements for comparing the organization's performance with internal past performance, the performance of other organizations, and with information from the literature (for example, practice guidelines, benchmarking)

____ The appropriateness of various technologies

____ The costs of various technologies

____ The need to support customer and supplier relationships

____ The analysis of resource use for patients with particular clinical problems to enhance the cost-effectiveness of care

____ The enhancement of work flow activity

____ The support needed for clinical and administrative decision making

____ The direction (for example, of library services, medical records, computer services) needed for the scope and complexity of services provided

Q. Do health care systems need to conduct systemwide management of information planning? What about health care networks? Should there be a networkwide plan? Should each organization in the network have a separate plan?

A. Although it may make sense for a health care system to conduct systemwide planning, Joint Commission standards do not address this issue. The Joint Commission provides a special survey package for health care systems. As part of this package, we offer a corporate orientation at the system headquarters and then survey each individual hospital in the system. However, we do not accredit the system as a whole; rather, we accredit each hospital within that system.

Therefore, if a health care system decides to have a systemwide plan for the management of information, it should ensure that each hospital within that system has its own plan in place that is unique to that facility.

The answer is the opposite for health care networks. The Joint Commission views a network as an integrated provider of health care, which is composed of a central office and several adjunct providers (for example, hospitals, nursing homes, home care organizations, individual physician offices). During this type of survey, the Joint Commission renders one accreditation decision for the entire network.

The approach to the management of information in a network should be integrated and coordinated throughout the entire network. Surveyors will closely examine the systems you have in place for connecting and linking information among the various components and providers (for example, how does the home care organization transmit information to the hospital? Are data definitions uniform across the network?) Therefore, management of information planning should be done on a networkwide basis. Each individual component of the network may also choose to have its own management of information plan that reflects the networkwide approach.

Q. How often are organizations expected to reassess their information needs and/or revise their information plans?
A. The standards do not specifically address the reassessment of information management needs. IM.1 simply states that "information management needs are based on a comprehensive assessment of needs." Since needs are expected to change, organizations should consider how they plan to continually reassess

them. Any good plan includes a mechanism designed for measuring and assessing the implementation of that plan. Typically, organizational policy defines how frequently plans are reviewed (for example, annually, revise as needed). An organization might identify priorities as part of the initial needs assessment and then establish measures and mechanisms to continually assess how well it is achieving those priorities. The management of information plan should be revised as needed over time.

Over the next few years, surveyors will be primarily concerned with whether or not an initial assessment was conducted. However, as organizations are resurveyed under these standards, the issue of reassessment may arise.

Q. Which staff members should be involved in the planning?
A. Because the management of information is an organization-wide function that affects all staff members, as well as external users, the planning approach should be multidisciplinary. Standard IM.1 emphasizes the necessity of considering the needs of individuals or groups whom the function serves or will serve. This includes, for example, governance, managers, clinical staff, inpatients and ambulatory patients, patients' families, payers and purchasers, regulatory bodies, and accreditation bodies.

The level of each of these individuals' or groups' involvement in the various aspects of planning will vary. Some (for example, chief information officer, medical record professionals) should be intimately involved in all aspects of planning. Other users might only be interviewed or consulted about their current and future information needs. For example, the chief information officer might talk to payers to assess whether they are receiving the information they need.

Some individuals or groups might be brought in on a consultative basis when needed. For example, when assessing and selecting interactive management of information systems for clinical and organizational information, a task force might be assigned that includes members of the medical staff, nurses, and other caregivers.

Q. Will surveyors audit our information system? Will they expect a demonstration of any information technology we use?
A. No. They will not do an audit of your records and/or databases (for example, audit trails). As described in more detail in Chapter 3, surveyors will review the documents that describe planning activities, interview key individuals involved in information planning, and talk to staff members. At certain points in the process, surveyors might ask to see specific records, reports, or files that relate to particular requirements. For example, they might ask to see a list of standard data elements (IM.3) or your organization's poison-control information (IM.9.5).

Surveyors will be looking to understand your processes for managing different types of information and how well those processes enhance the delivery of quality patient care. If your organization is significantly computerized, you might find it easier to describe these processes to the surveyor(s) by, for example, pulling up different reports on a screen or demonstrating how a physician might access a computerized patient record. However, the surveyors' main concern is the performance of your information management processes—that is, are users receiving the right information, at the right time, and in the right manner?

Q. Is a request for proposal (RFP) *evidence of information management planning*?
A. No. The acquisition of computer technology is only one part of an organization's planning activities, and should typically occur after an intensive assessment period. The Joint Commission is more interested in what happened before you decided to issue an RFP. What systems do you anticipate this equipment being a part of? What needs is this computer system

going to fulfill? Who was involved in assessing and selecting the computer system? Again, the Joint Commission considers technology to be only a tool for carrying out effective information management. The Joint Commission is more concerned about the management of information *processes* that the tool(s) supports and how those processes impact the delivery of patient care.

APPLICATION EXAMPLE 1.

Approaching a Needs Assessment

Standard IM.1 requires that the management of information processes be "planned and designed to meet the health care organization's internal and external information needs." In approaching this standard, organizations might ask:
- What are our internal and external information needs, both now and in the future?
- How well are we meeting or planning to meet those needs?
- What do we need to do differently to meet those needs?
- Or to put it another way: Where are we now and where do we need to be?

As detailed in the scoring guidelines for IM.1, organizations are expected to conduct a comprehensive assessment of information needs upon which they can base their information planning. This requirement reflects the first two boxes in the Joint Commission's cycle within the framework for improving performance (see Figure 2, page 20). Before organizations can design management of information processes, staff members need to determine specific objectives that guide the effort.

Given the volume of information that passes through a health care organization on an average day, conducting a needs assessment is not an easy task. It involves the following:
- Determining the different types of information required by different individuals and groups (for example, patient-based, aggregate data);

- Assessing whether the proper processes are in place to manage this information (for example, data capture, data transmission);
- Determining whether users have access to the information they need within the required time frame to carry out various activities (for example, inpatient care activities, in research);
- Determining whether users know how to use the data or information they request and/or require;
- Considering how data needs might change in the future; and
- Setting priorities.

Depending on the size and complexity of your organization, an initial needs assessment could take a few months to a year.

Organizations can take various approaches to assessing their information needs. As indicated earlier, Joint Commission requirements encourage organizations to develop creative approaches to meeting the standards. The following paragraphs offer some tips on how organizations might approach this endeavor.

Form a Multidisciplinary Team

Because the management of information is an organizational function that affects the majority of staff members, organizational leaders might consider forming a multidisciplinary task force or team. This task force might conduct the needs assessment, set priorities for improvement, and oversee the design or redesign of projects. Members might include the administrator; chief information officer; medical staff chairperson; attending and house staff; and directors of admitting, patient accounts, laboratory, nursing, quality improvement, risk management, utilization management, and health information management. Eventually, the task force might want to assign subteams or representatives to conduct various aspects of the needs assessment.

Some task forces have set objectives or visions. For example, the Information Management Council at Dixie Regional Medical

Center, a 107-bed hospital in St. George, Utah, defined a mission and vision statement with specific objectives for the council (see Table 3, page 34). When the council was first organized, "the concept of information management was new enough to all of us [the council] that we were uncertain how to proceed." The vision and mission statement helped focus the council's activities.[1]

The Standards as a Guide

The standards provide a framework for assessing and planning your organization's processes for managing information. Based on accepted principles of the management of information, IM.1 through IM.6 explain the fundamental issues that need to be considered when managing information. The task force might refer to the flowchart of the standards (see Figure 1, page 12) to guide its efforts. This flowchart essentially provides a *macroview* of what your processes for managing information should include.

In addition, the scoring guidelines for IM.1.1 provide an extensive list of items that organizations need to consider when conducting a needs assessment, including support needed for planning purposes; requirements for internal and external transmission of data or information; and longitudinal data or information reporting needs (see Table 2, page 27). This list should prove useful when conducting an assessment. However, organizations should customize this list to their own needs. There may be additional items you'll want to consider, or some of the items may be irrelevant to your organization.

Determine How Information Is Currently Managed

Inventory the different types of data and information (that is, patient-based, aggregate, knowledge-based, comparative). For

---

[1] Thomason M: Implementing the new Joint Commission information management standards: One hospital's approach. Journal of AHIMA, 65 (5):66–67, May 1994.

TABLE 3 Sample Information Management Statement of Purpose

Vision
The purpose of good management is to ensure appropriate, timely decisions and actions to render improved services. Correct decisions hinge on information; therefore, the Information Management Council resolves to provide and interpret information to assist the hospital's vision to become the best 100-bed hospital in America.

Mission
To enhance the decision making of clinical and management users, and to assist in quantifying quality of service and quality of gains, the Information Management Council (IMC) will ensure that the provision of information is:
- Accurate
- Timely
- Meaningful
- Objective

To reach this objective, the IMC will be responsible for:

1. Setting standards for data collection, processing, and reporting. This will take the form of policy statements, as well as requiring data collection departments to have clear and consistent procedures for data collection.
2. Monitoring and assessing data quality by routine quality audits, as well as data comparisons with external sources.
3. Planning and reporting for projects that involve intradepartment information collection.
4. Drafting a coordinated plan for allocations of resources available. Reviewing funds and participating in recommendations for purchases of systems or software to meet Dixie Regional Medical Center's information needs.
5. Assessing the needs of information users, to make sure that existing reporting is accurate, timely, meaningful, and objective. Develop a tool (Report Request Form) to assist users in clearly identifying their information needs.
6. Ensuring confidentiality of information. Developing standard policies for release of information and security, which is not limited to computerized information.
7. Assisting in quality assessment. Helping departments to measure the quality of patient services by assisting them in determining their needs for data collection and reporting.

Source: Dixie Regional Medical Center, St. George, Utah. Reprinted with permission.

each type of information, a member or subgroup of the task force might conduct an inventory. You'll want to look for data dynasties. These can occur when information is gathered, analyzed, and used in areas of an organization without the knowledge of all interested parties. Efficiencies in data-collection activities and opportunities to share information go unnoticed if staff are unaware of their colleagues' activities. (See section on IM.3, page 186, for additional advice on conducting a data and information inventory.)

Determine If You're Meeting Users' Needs

The task force might identify the different users of information (for example by job category or affiliation—leaders, department managers, medical staff). This should include the identification of external and internal users. The task force might then develop a survey for each user group. Questions might focus on whether users are getting the information they need in the time frame required to effectively carry out various activities. In determining interview questions, organizations should consider the three questions posed in Chapter 1:

- *Are internal and external users receiving the right information?* This question focuses on the accuracy of the information that users receive (that is, are they receiving what they asked for?) as well as the efficacy and appropriateness of that information (that is, is the information relevant? Has it been shown to accomplish its desired end?). For example, organizations might ask physicians if they are receiving the lab reports they request. That is, if they order a complete blood count on a patient, are they receiving the results of a complete blood count? Or you might ask leaders if the monthly financial reports they receive are useful in making decisions and setting strategies. If not, you might ask what information would be useful.
- *Are users receiving this information in a manner in which they need it?* This question asks whether the coordination of information

among users is adequate and whether the format in which that information is presented is effective. For example, is your organization able to compile the information requested by the comparative database to which you belong? Are you able to provide that information in the format that the database requests? Do all caregivers feel that the format of the patient record is conducive to making patient care decisions?

- *Are users receiving information when they need it?* This question deals with access to information and the timeliness in which that information is received. It asks whether users are able to obtain the information they need to carry out patient care, research, and other activities and whether that information is available when they need it—not two hours or two days late. For example, can a home care nurse count on having the complete patient record available before she visits a patient for the first time? Can a team that is developing a practice guideline for total hip-replacement patients obtain relevant and up-to-date literature between meetings? Can a physician access necessary information concerning adverse drug reactions before prescribing a medication?

As shown in Table 4, page 37, these questions relate directly to the Joint Commission's nine dimensions of performance: efficacy, appropriateness, availability, effectiveness, timeliness, safety, efficiency, continuity, and respect and caring. These dimensions strongly affect patient outcomes and resource use. Organizations can use these dimensions in assessing the performance of the different functions within the accreditation manuals. (Note: Some of these dimensions are not relevant to the management of certain types of information.)

Determine Priorities

Once internal and external needs are identified, an organization needs to set priorities for improvement. In other words, what is working well? What is not? What is most important to fix now? What resources are involved? One way to set priorities is to

TABLE 4 Dimensions of Performance

The Right Information

Efficacy: The degree to which data and information used in processes has been shown to accomplish the desired or projected outcome(s).

Appropriateness: The degree to which the data and information provided is relevant to users' needs, given the state of the art.

Provided at the Right Time

Availability: The degree to which appropriate data and information is available to meet the needs of users.

Timeliness: The degree to which the data and information is provided at the time it is most beneficial or necessary.

Provided in the Right Manner

Effectiveness: The degree to which the data and information is provided in the correct manner, given the current state of the art, to achieve the desired or projected outcome.

Continuity: The degree to which data and information is coordinated among users, among organizations, and across time.

Safety: The degree to which data and information reduces the risk of an intervention and risk in the care environment.

Efficiency: The ratio of the outcomes (results) to the data and information resources used to obtain these results.

Respect and Caring: The degree to which a patient, or designee, is involved in his or her own information-based care decisions, and that those providing data and information do so with sensitivity and respect for his or her needs, expectations, and individual differences.

divide needs into three categories: *must have, need,* and *wish we had*. Once objectives are set, the organization might develop a plan and assign different task forces to accomplish these objectives. These task forces might consider the use of applicable information technology as a way to simplify certain processes.

Confidentiality, Security, and Integrity of Information (IM.2–IM.2.3)

RELATED STANDARDS

IM.2 *The information-management function provides for information confidentiality, security, and integrity.*

IM.2.1 (Capped at Score 3)
A 1 2 3 4 5 NA The organization determines the need for and appropriate levels of security and confidentiality of data and information.

IM.2.2 (Capped at Score 4)
A 1 2 3 4 5 NA The organization determines how data and information can be retrieved on a timely and easy basis without compromising the data's and information's security and confidentiality.

IM.2.2.1 (Capped at Score 3)
A 1 2 3 4 5 NA A written organizational and medical staff policy requires that medical records may be removed from the organization's jurisdiction and safekeeping only in accordance with a court order, subpoena, or statute.

IM.2.2.2 (Capped at Score 4)
A 1 2 3 4 5 NA The organization has a functioning mechanism designed to preserve the confidentiality of data and information identified as sensitive or requiring extraordinary means to protect patient privacy.

IM.2.3 (No cap)
A 1 2 3 4 5 NA The organization has a functioning mechanism designed to safeguard records and information

against loss, destruction, tampering, and unauthorized access or use.

AN OVERVIEW OF REQUIREMENTS

The necessity of maintaining the proper balance between data access and data confidentiality has been much discussed in recent literature, particularly with the advent of the computerized patient record. The intent for IM.2–IM.2.3 states that an effective process for determining appropriate levels of confidentiality identifies at least:

- Who has access to information;
- The information to which an individual has access;
- The obligation of the individual who has access to information to keep it confidential;
- Policies regarding release of health information and/or removal of the medical record; and
- The mechanism designed to secure information against unauthorized intrusion, corruption, and damage.

None of these requirements, which appeared in the former "Medical Records" chapter, is new. However, the standards are now broader. Organizations are now required to assess the need for confidentiality, security, and integrity of all types of data and information, not just patient and billing information.

■ How Are These Standards Surveyed?

Surveyors will assess how well an organization maintains confidentiality and security of information by reviewing documents, interviewing staff who access information, and making observations. For example, the surveyors will examine any policies and documents related to the security and confidentiality of data and information, removal of information from the organization, and safeguarding records and information against loss, destruction, and tampering. During the management of information interview, the surveyor will ask appropriate individuals to describe what measures are in place to ensure confidentiality, security, and integrity of information. They will also verify whether or not your organization is complying with local, state, and federal confidentiality and/or privacy regulations, laws, and statutes. Questions regarding these standards may also be asked during other interview sessions or visits to patient care settings.

Because the management of information is an organization-wide function, an organization's compliance with these standards will become evident during the course of the survey. Surveyors will observe how well your processes work as they review other standards in the *AMH*. For example, when assessing standards related to the "Continuum of Care" chapter, surveyors might establish by observation if the appropriate balance between access and confidentiality is maintained when sharing data and information among different providers.

COMMON QUESTIONS

Q. What is considered an appropriate level of security and confidentiality?
A. It depends on the type of information as well as applicable laws and organizational policy. Some data are more sensitive and require a higher level of confidentiality than others. For example, patient-specific data will often require a higher level of confidentiality than knowledge-based data. In addition, certain types of patient data (for example, related to substance abuse) would be considered extra sensitive and require a very high level of confidentiality. It is up to your organization to define what an appropriate level of confidentiality is for different types of information.

You might begin by determining which levels of confidentiality are necessary for different types of information (for example, high, low, none). Then, you might determine who should be given access to what information. This could be done according to job title, responsibilities, and/or function. Organizations should also develop policies and procedures regarding the release of sensitive information to external bodies or removal of the medical record from the organization. Once all these factors are taken into account, you can design the appropriate mechanism(s) for securing confidentiality.

Q. What would the Joint Commission consider an effective mechanism for ensuring confidentiality?
A. The particular mechanism(s) used to maintain confidentiality should be defined by the organization. Again, the Joint Commission is more interested in whether the mechanism(s) chosen is appropriate for the type of information being protected. There are different ways to protect confidentiality. Access to computer files can be controlled through security codes or by restricting certain operations to particular terminals. For example, the computer terminals in the finance department might only be accessed by individuals in that department and only to perform financial transactions. Manual mechanisms for maintaining confidentiality include locked cabinets or files for impaired physician information, specific medical records for psychiatry diagnoses, sign-out procedures, and hard copy medical records maintained in a secure, restricted-access location. Table 5, page 42, provides some sample security mechanisms.

Q. Besides patient care information, what other types of information might require confidentiality and security?
A. As described above, the main change to these requirements in 1994 was that organizations need to protect confidentiality for all types of information. Currently, most organizations have mechanisms in place designed to maintain confidentiality and security of patient care and billing data and information. However, health care organizations also house other types of data and information that may be considered sensitive or private, such as the following:

TABLE 5 Examples of Technical Security Features

User identification and authentication: Programs and procedures that (a) assign unique identification to each individual user of a system and (b) check information to verify the identity of the user.

Passwords: The most commonly used means of authentication, a password is information known only by the user it authenticates (and possibly by the security manager). Effective password procedures emphasize the use of character strings other than dictionary words, require passwords that are six or more characters long, and mandate new passwords periodically.

Access control mechanisms: Ways of automatically enforcing rules about which individuals and groups can access programs and data. Under **mandatory access control,** the most-sensitive resources are available only to persons cleared for access and with a specific need to do so; these persons cannot grant access to others who are not cleared. Under **discretionary access control,** owners of data and programs may grant access to others who have the need.

Encryption: Alteration of information so that it cannot be understood if it is received or accessed by unauthorized persons. Encryption is used to store particularly sensitive information such as passwords or to protect information being transmitted over nonsecure channels.

Audit log: A record of actions performed on data by users that potentially could violate the security policy of a system (for example, log-ons, file accesses). Audit logs may
(a) help detect breaches of confidentiality;
(b) deter authorized users from accessing data for which they have no need; and
(c) demonstrate, if there is a breach, that an organization properly safeguarded the automated data.

Transaction log: A record of changes to data, especially to a database, that can be used to reconstruct the data if there is a failure after the transaction occurs. Transaction logs are a means of ensuring data integrity and availability.

Backup and recovery mechanisms: Techniques, such as maintaining redundant systems or applying transaction logs, that enable a system to return to operation after a failure or catastrophe.

Dial-back modems: A means of authenticating a user who calls in to access a system by calling the user back at a predetermined phone number.

Security guards, gateways, intelligent routers: Computers and software dedicated to protecting networks or subnetworks. These devices authenticate outside users before allowing them any access to the network. They can be effective in securing networks that have Internet or other general-purpose external connections.

Source: Lawrence L: Safeguarding the confidentiality of automated medical information. *Joint Commission Journal on Quality Improvement* 20:639–646, Nov 1994.

- *Human resource-related information.* Certain information about staff members (for example, medical history) may be considered private.
- *Peer review and/or credentialing information.* Most health care organizations have mechanisms to ensure confidentiality of this type of information.
- *Practitioner-specific data used in performance-improvement activities and credentialing.* In these instances, the practitioners' identities are typically kept confidential.
- *Research information, which belongs to the grantor.*
- *Proprietary source codes for information systems.* The source codes are property of the vendor and must be kept confidential by the user hospital.
- *Risk management data regarding potential and current liabilities, such as information focusing on malpractice claims.*
- *Strategic planning documents, for competitive reasons.*

Again, organizations should conduct an inventory of the different types of information that pass through the organization. The sensitivity of each type of information should be considered and appropriate levels of confidentiality ensured.

Q. What is considered timely and easy retrieval of information?

A. Most standards under IM.2 address the protection and safeguarding of data and information. Standard IM.2.2 addresses the other side of the equation—access. Both issues are equally important in that caregivers need easy access to a variety of information to perform their jobs. Yet, organizations also have an obligation to protect the privacy of patients and others. The organizations must protect confidentiality and provide for appropriate access. It's a balancing act, and the Joint Commission's standards focus on your organization's ability to maintain the proper balance. That is, are practitioners able to retrieve all parts of the medical record when they need it? And, at the same time, is the patient's confidentiality secured?

In most instances, the Joint Commission leaves it up to the organization to define "timely and easy access." The definition will differ for various types of information. Obviously, caregivers need more immediate access to the medical record than to aggregate data for performance-improvement activities. In defining what timely and easy access is for different types of information, you should consult with the different users of information in your organization.

Q. What type of information is considered sensitive and requires extraordinary protection?
A. As discussed earlier, certain types of information are more sensitive than others. This typically applies to patient-specific information (for example, information related to the diagnosis or treatment of certain psychiatric disorders, substance abuse, AIDS). Certain portions of the medical record may be so confidential that organizations need to take extraordinary means to preserve a patient's privacy. For example, an organization might store sensitive portions of the medical record separately from the rest of the record. Other types of data and information requiring extraordinary protection include risk management or peer review data; information related to employee health such as occupational exposure to needle sticks or HIV testing; and human resource information such as payroll or salary figures.

Even when information is highly sensitive, organizations need to maintain a balance between confidentiality and access. Appropriate staff members should be able to access this information when necessary for medical care or follow-up, review functions, or use in performance-improvement activities.

Q. Does an organization's policy concerning the removal of information need to cover all types of information?
A. No. The standard covers only patient-specific information. Your organization should have a policy stating that medical records may only be removed from the organization's

jurisdiction and safekeeping in accordance with a court order, subpoena, or statute. However, your organization might want to consider expanding this policy, or developing additional policies that cover the removal of other types of information such as risk management or malpractice claims data.

Q. How can an organization ensure data security and integrity during the transition from a manual system to a computer system?
A. The Joint Commission realizes that, over the next several years, many organizations will be making a transition from a manual to a computerized patient record. You may also be computerizing other processes (for example, credentialing) or changing from one type of computer system to another (for example, mainframe to local area networks). Although the Joint Commission recognizes the challenges of such a transition, you are still expected to ensure the security and integrity of information within these systems.

During these transitions, organizations must ensure that backup provisions are in place when critical applications are being moved to different environments.

Q. What will surveyors look for in a disaster recovery plan?
A. Surveyors will check that your organization planned for the recovery of important data and information in the event of a disaster (for example, theft, vandalism, loss of critical data, provision of emergency power, and fire and flood recovery). This might be documented in policies and procedures, meeting minutes, a management of information plan, or a separate disaster recovery plan. Disaster recovery planning might be completed as part of your organization's overall information planning activities. As the different types of information are identified, you might prioritize whatever information is important and needs to be saved in case of disaster, as appropriate for the size and complexity of the organization.

The manner in which information is safeguarded depends on the type of information. For example, electronic information can be routinely backed up and stored elsewhere. Storage of paper documents will depend on the reproducibility of documents. Some documents of historical value cannot be reproduced and should be stored permanently off-site, for example. The type of storage used also depends on how often you have to access the information. For example, archival information that is rarely used (for example, solely for research) might be stored in a vault.

Uniform Data Definitions and Methods for Capturing Data (IM.3–IM.3.3)

RELATED STANDARDS

IM.3 *When feasible, uniform data definitions and methods for capturing data are in place.*

IM.3.1 (Capped at Score 2)
A 1 2 3 4 5 NA Whenever possible, minimum data sets, data definitions, codes, classifications, and terminology are standardized throughout the organization.

IM.3.1.1 (Capped at Score 2)
A 1 2 3 4 5 NA The organization references externally standardized sets, definitions, codes, classifications, and terminology (when available) when developing its organization standards.

IM.3.2 (Capped at Score 3)
A 1 2 3 4 5 NA The organization collects data in a timely, economical, and efficient manner and with the degree of accuracy, completeness, and discrimination necessary for their intended use.

IM.3.3 (Capped at Score 2)

A 1 2 3 4 5 NA   The organization implements mechanisms designed to ascertain that bias in the data is minimized and to assess the data's reliability, validity, and accuracy on an ongoing basis.

AN OVERVIEW OF REQUIREMENTS

These standards ask that you speak and use the same information "language," at least within your own organization and as much as possible with others in the health care field. This means that, whenever feasible, uniform data definitions and methods for capturing data should be in place. This requirement ties in closely with the "Improving Organizational Performance" chapter. With standardized terminology, definitions, and data-collection methods, organizations will be able to compare performance across departments or with other organizations.

Whenever possible, organizations should standardize the following:

- Uniform data definitions—an agreed upon and accepted set of terms and definitions. Examples include policies and procedures to address data collection and usage, a data dictionary, or a quality-control system for data collection and entry.
- Minimum data sets—an agreed upon and accepted set of terms and definitions for whatever constitutes a collection (or set) of related data items. Examples include Uniform Hospital Discharge Data Set (UHDDS), Uniform Clinical Data Set (UCDS), and Medical Subject Headings (MESH).
- Codes and classification systems—a grouping of related entities to produce necessary statistical information such as diagnostic-related groups (DRGs).

- Nomenclature—a recognized system of preferred terminology for naming disease processes. Examples include the International Classification of Diseases—9th Edition—Clinical Modification (ICD-9-CM), Current Procedural Terminology (CPT), Systematized Nomenclature of Pathology (SNOP), and the Nursing Interventions Classification from the University of Iowa.
- Uniform abbreviations—Organizations should ensure that all departments and staff use the same abbreviations (for example, KVO means keep vein open; OUT means out of town; and SOB means shortness of breath).

Organizations can typically conduct an inventory of data sets, terminology, and nomenclature at the same time they conduct an assessment of management of information needs. (Figure 3, page 49, provides a form that organizations might use to conduct such an inventory.) At this time, organizations should be on the lookout for data dynasties. Also, staff members in a department might be labeling information with the same name but plugging in different data for each. For example, "admission type" may be used to mean different things in various departments. Organizations might want to develop a data dictionary (Figure 4, page 50) when standardizing their terminology and consider using national and state guidelines for data set uniformity and connectivity, as available, and any other external guides such as those found in the Uniform Bill 92 (UB92).

Organizations also need to ensure that their systems for capturing data are effective, timely, and economical. For example, are statistically appropriate sampling procedures defined? Are there defined criteria for data capture and data input? Mechanisms should be in place to minimize data bias and to assess the reliability, validity, and accuracy of data on an ongoing basis.

■ How Are These Standards Surveyed?

During the document review session, surveyors will review any policies, standards, or procedures an organization has relating

FIGURE 3 Sample Form for Data Inventory

Database Inventory Part I: Health Information Management
                                   _____
                                        (Name of Department)

Instructions: List below all logs, records, files, and information systems that are maintained in your department. For each, indicate whether the data is maintained in a manual or automated* system and the period of time for which the database is maintained.

Database Name	Automated	Dates	Manual	Dates
Disease Operation Index	X	1961–present	X	1933–1960
Physicians Index	X	1961–present	X	1933–1960
Abstract	X	1972–present		
Master Patient Index	X	1983–present	X	1922–1982
Analysis of Hospital Service Statistics	X	1986–present	X	1972–1985
Death Log	X	1984–present	X	1964–1983
Correspondence Log			X	1985–present
Subpoena Log			X	1985–present
ER Log			X	1960–present
OR Log			X	1968–present
Admission, Discharge, Transfer Lists			X	1961–present
Census Reports			X	1987–present

*Automated databases are those capable of electronic retrieval.

When conducting a needs assessment, organizations might use a form similar to this one to complete a data inventory.

FIGURE 4 Data Dictionary

Data Element	Element Description
Hospital Newborn	Patient was born in this hospital. Calculated by admit type on admission and from service at discharge. Space = No, 1 = Yes
ICU Days	Number of days on ICU unit for adults; identified through US 82 revenue codes. Excludes discharge day.
Inout Code	1 = Inpatient, 0 = Outpatient
Ins Returned Outlier	DRG code, as determined by Medicare, sent at time of payment. Access Code Table "DRG" in Transition 1 for transition.
Ins Returned Outlier	Outlier status, as determined by Medicare, sent at time of payment. 1 = Day Outlier, 2= Cost Outlier
Last Discharge Date	Discharge date of patient's previous visit to hospital in YYMMDD format.
Leave Begin Date	Date patient went on leave in YYMMDD format.
Leave Days	Number of days on leave calculated by leave and date minus leave begin date.
Leave End Date	Date patient returned from leave in YYMMDD format.
Length of Stay	Length of stay (discharge date – admission date – any leave days). If admitted and discharged on same day, value will be 1. Only applies to inpatient.
Marital Status	Patient's marital status code and transition. Access Code Table "MRS" in Transition 1 for transition.
MDC	Major diagnostic category associated with Medical DRG; assigned to all Inpatients. Access Code Table "MDC" in Transition 1 for transition.
Med Surg Days	Days on medical/surgical unit. Determined through US 82 revenue codes. Excludes discharge day.

Above are examples of data definitions to enable staff in an organization to "speak the same language."

FIGURE 4 Data Dictionary *(continued)*

Source	Field Size	Timing	Used to Search Y/N	Coded Field Y/N	Module
Hospital Calculated	1	Admission Abstract	Yes	No	COM
Hospital Calculated	3	Billing	Yes	No	COM
Admitting	1	Admission	Yes	No	COM
Medicare	3	Payment	No	Yes	COM
Medicare	1	Payment	No	No	COM
Hospital Calculated	6	Admission	No	No	COM
Nsg Unit	6	During Stay	No	No	COM
Hospital Calculated	3	During Stay	No	No	COM
Nsg Unit	6	During Stay	No	No	COM
Hospltal Calculated	4	Discharge	Yes	No	COM
Admitting	1	Admission	No	Yes	COM
Hospital Calculated	2	Abstract	Yes	Yes	COM
Hospital Calculated	3	Billing	Yes	No	COM

to uniform data definitions and uniform methods for capturing data. Later, a surveyor will hold an interview with key staff members involved in the management of information. At that time, the surveyor will ask about what uniform data definitions and methods for capturing data are in place. As they tour the organization, surveyors might also ask questions related to this topic. For example, in the medical records department, the surveyor might inquire about the coding systems you use. On a patient unit, the surveyor might ask a staff member to describe how charges are captured.

Most of these standards (IM.3.1, IM.3.1.1, and IM.3.3) are capped at a Score of 2. Thus, organizations have a few years to achieve compliance with these requirements. However, standardizing data definitions, nomenclature, and the like should probably be one of the first steps in developing organization-wide processes for managing information. Without uniform data definitions, organizations would have difficulty meeting the rest of the standards in this chapter. Therefore, your organization might want to make standardization an early priority in management of information planning.

IM.3.2, which deals with data collection, is capped at a Score of 3. If your organization receives worse than a score of 2 on this standard, it could result in a type 1 recommendation.

COMMON QUESTIONS

Q. In determining data definitions, should national and state definitions take precedence over organizational definitions?
A. Although Joint Commission standards do not address this directly, the reasonable response would be yes. As stated in the intent for IM.3–IM.3.3, these standards are intended to "facilitate comparisons of data and information within and among organizations..." If you give your own local definitions priority, you will not be able to externally benchmark how you compare

to other organizations. Thus, you should consider existing external definitions. Some definitions are required by external agencies (for example, Medicare billing), while others are offered merely as guidelines (for example, the Joint Commission's IMSystem indicator definitions or the Center for Disease Control's definitions of infection).

Q. Who is responsible for setting data definitions?
A. The standards do not assign direct responsibility for this activity to a particular person or job classification. Ultimately, the Joint Commission views organizational leaders as responsible for the entire management of information function, as well as the other important functions in the *AMH*. Typically, however, this responsibility would be assigned to an information management director, medical records director, or another appropriate person.

Q. What does the Joint Commission mean by "timely" data collection?
A. Typically, the Joint Commission does not define time frames for collecting data, but there are some instances when we do. For example, the assessment of a patient admitted to a hospital must be completed within 24 hours. This requirement is an exception, since time frames are otherwise determined by the particular organization. When determining what "timely" collection is for different types of information, organizations should consider the users' needs and the potential impact on patient care.

Q. Does the Joint Commission require any particular mechanisms for assessing bias, reliability, validity, or accuracy?
A. No. Once again, the particular method for meeting the intent of standard IM.3.3 is left to the organization to determine.

Medical Record Review (IM.3.3.1–IM.3.3.1.2)

RELATED STANDARDS

IM.3.3.1 (Not capped)

A 1 2 3 4 5 NA The organization reviews the completeness, accuracy, and timely completion of information in medical records at least quarterly.

IM.3.3.1.1 (Capped at Score 4)

A 1 2 3 4 5 NA The review is performed by, at a minimum, the medical staff in cooperation with nursing, the health information-management (medical record) service, management and administrative services, and representatives of other departments as appropriate.

IM.3.3.1.2 (Capped at Score 4)

A 1 2 3 4 5 NA The review determines that each medical record, or a representative sample of records, reflects the diagnosis, diagnostic test results, therapy, the patient's condition and in-hospital progress, and the patient's condition at discharge.

AN OVERVIEW OF REQUIREMENTS

Organizations must review a representative sample of medical records on at least a quarterly basis. Essentially, the Joint Commission is concerned whether or not documentation supports the therapy or other care provided to the patient. The purpose of this review is to ensure the completeness, accuracy, and timely completion of the record. This review should be based on predefined criteria, which are focused on the quality of the documentation.

The scoring guidelines include a list of items that all completed medical records should contain (see Table 6, below). Organizations might want to use this list to develop criteria specific to their own organizations or for specific conditions.

TABLE 6 Checklist for Quarterly Medical Record Review

The following is addressed in a representative sample of records:
Check all that apply.

- ____ Identification data
- ____ Medical history, including the chief complaint; details of the present illness; relevant past, social, and family histories (appropriate to the patient's age); and an inventory by body system
- ____ A summary of the patient's psychosocial needs, as appropriate to the patient's age
- ____ A report of relevant physical examinations
- ____ A statement on the conclusions or impressions drawn from the admission history and physical examination
- ____ A statement on the course of action planned for the patient for this episode of care and of its periodic review, as appropriate
- ____ Diagnostic and therapeutic orders
- ____ Evidence of appropriate informed consent
- ____ Clinical observations, including the results of therapy
- ____ Progress notes made by the medical staff and other authorized staff
- ____ Consultation reports
- ____ Reports of operative and other invasive procedures, tests, and their results
- ____ Reports of any diagnostic and therapeutic procedures, such as pathology and clinical laboratory examinations and radiology and nuclear medicine examinations or treatments
- ____ Records of donation and receipt of transplants and/or implants
- ____ Final diagnosis(es)
- ____ Conclusions at termination of hospitalization
- ____ Clinical resumes and discharge summaries
- ____ Discharge instructions to the patient and/or family
- ____ Results of autopsy, when performed

These requirements are not new; the standards were previously scored under the "Medical Staff" chapter because they were viewed primarily as the responsibility of the medical staff. Now, the activity is recognized as an organizational responsibility, not just a medical staff responsibility.

■ How Are These Standards Surveyed?

During the document review session, surveyors will review any policies and procedures your organization has relating to the content of the patient record, and its completeness, accuracy, and timely completion. They will also review and evaluate your organization's last four quarterly medical record reviews. During the medical record interview, surveyors will ask staff members to describe how they conduct their periodic record reviews. (See Chapter 3 for a more complete description of the survey process for these standards.)

Since these are existing requirements, none of these standards are capped. Therefore, your organization could receive a type 1 recommendation if you score 3 or worse on these standards.

COMMON QUESTIONS

Q. What is meant by a multidisciplinary review? Is this a new requirement?
A. A multidisciplinary review of the medical record should include representatives from nursing, the medical staff, administration, and information management. The standards have always required representatives from these four groups to participate in a multidisciplinary review. However, now that medical record review is recognized as an organizational responsibility, rather than primarily a medical staff responsibility, the multidisciplinary nature of this review is more greatly emphasized. It is appropriate to expand the participation, perhaps on a rotating basis, to other caregivers (for example, dietitians, physical therapists, social workers) and to include their documentation in the medical record review.

Q. What is considered a representative sample for review?
A. The sample of medical records chosen for review should represent the practitioners providing care and the types of care provided in an organization or in a department or service. It should encompass the full scope of practice, including the most common diagnoses and procedures and all high-risk procedures.

Q. Is the review expected to be performed on an organizationwide or department-specific basis?
A. Either is fine. It depends on your organization's policies and preferences. If the review is done on an organizationwide basis, the sample used should be representative of the scope of practice across the organization. If it is done on a departmental basis, the sample should be representative of the department's scope of practice. If departmentalized, data should be shared among departments to ensure comparability of documentation for similar types of records.

Q. How often should medical records from each physician be reviewed?
A. The medical records of each physician on your medical staff should be reviewed at least annually.

Q. When is a medical record considered delinquent?
A. A medical record is defined as "delinquent" if it has not been completed within a hospital-defined time period following patient discharge. This time period should be specified in the medical staff's rules and regulations and, from the Joint Commission's perspective, may not exceed 30 days. Hospital staff and medical staff should collaborate to complete medical records as soon after discharge as possible so that information can promptly be retrieved for clinical, legal, or performance improvement purposes. According to Joint Commission guidelines, a type I recommendation is attached to the accreditation decision if any of the following situations exist:

- The total number of medical records delinquent for any reason exceeds 50% of the average monthly discharges (AMD). A score of 3 is given when the number of delinquent medical records is 50% to 74% of the AMD; a score of 4 when the number of delinquent medical records is 75% to 99% of the AMD; and a score of 5 when the total number of delinquent medical records is greater than the AMD.
- The number of medical records that are delinquent due to the absence of a medical history and physical examination exceeds nine records or 2% of the AMD, whichever is greater.
- The number of medical records delinquent due to the absence of an operative report exceeds nine records or 2% of the average monthly operative procedures, whichever is greater.

Education and Training of Staff (IM.4)

RELATED STANDARD

IM.4 (Capped at Score 3)

 A 1 2 3 4 5 NA Decision makers and other individuals in the organization who generate, collect, and analyze data and information are educated and trained in the principles of information management.

AN OVERVIEW OF REQUIREMENTS

For information to be managed effectively, the individuals involved in the generation, collection, analysis, and use of data and information must be educated and trained in such areas as using measurement instruments or statistical tools, collecting unbiased data, and/or using data and information to help make decisions. The training and education provided should reflect individual staff members' needs and responsibilities.

■ How Is This Standard Surveyed?

Surveyors will ask staff members who generate information or make use of it in their activities to describe the education they have had in the principles of management of information. The surveyor may also review any written materials related to management of information training and education, such as staff education outlines regarding the management of information, individual performance reports showing continuing education, reports and/or minutes documenting data analysis, and attendance reports combined with lecture outlines. This issue will be addressed as part of the organization's competency assessment process.

Organizations are not expected to fully train all appropriate staff in the management of information by 1995. A reasonable expectation over the next few years is for organizations to plan an approach that will ultimately meet the full intent of the standard. This plan should identify the education needs of different staff members (at least according to job categories), explain the plan for providing appropriate education to staff members, define priorities for implementation, and begin to implement the plan.

COMMON QUESTIONS

Q. Who is expected to be trained?
A. Anyone in your organization who generates, collects, analyzes, and/or uses data and information. Essentially, this means all staff. As stressed throughout this book, almost every staff person has some relationship to data and information, whether they collect admissions data from patients, use aggregate financial data to make purchasing decisions, or assess patient information to determine a diagnosis or treatment plan. Obviously, a

medical record clerk's relationship to data and information is different than an administrator's. And, the administrator's relationship is different from a nurse's or physician's. Thus, training needs of different staff vary. Some staff, such as admissions clerks, might only need "awareness training" that helps them understand their role in handling data and information. Others, such as administrators, might need more in-depth training.

Q. What does the Joint Commission expect leaders and staff to know about the management of information? What level of training should be provided to different staff?
A. As described in the previous question, staff should have the knowledge about and training on the management of information they need to carry out their responsibilities. For example, staff members who collect data or enter data into databases need to understand, at the least, the basics of data integrity. They need to understand the implications of accidentally transposing numbers, the necessity for accuracy checking, and so forth. Staff members who analyze data and assemble data reports need to have some basic statistical skills, such as how to design and read a control chart. Organizational leaders need to understand the limitations of the data and information they are working with before decisions based on that data are made. Therefore, they must have some understanding of statistics and variation. (See Application Example 2, page 62, for some tips on evaluating management of information training needs.)

Q. If an organization offers staff members a computer course, will this meet the intent of the standard?
A. Only if it covers management of information principles. Providing computer training is quickly becoming a necessity within many organizations as they automate various functions. Some computer courses simply focus on how to operate the hardware and software. This type of training would not meet the intent of the standards because it focuses only on how to use

a tool. It does not teach the underlying principles of the management of information, such as how to use data and information in decision making. For example, a staff member might be taught a computer program that can create a control chart. However, if he or she does not understand the underlying statistical principles governing this control chart, then his or her ability to use this chart in performance improvement activities will be limited.

There are ways to combine computer training with training in the management of information. Some organizations might decide to demonstrate principles of the management of information at the same time they train staff on a new information system. In this way, information technology becomes a tool to demonstrate the management of information.

Q. Who is responsible for overseeing the training of staff in the management of information?
A. The standards do not designate a particular person or department. The decision is left to the organization and should be determined as part of organizational planning activities. Some organizations may combine management of information training with other educational activities. The Joint Commission requires organizations to determine and address the educational needs of staff. This includes the many different types of education that staff members need and might logically encompass management of information training as well. Thus, an organization's education or human resources department might be made responsible for fulfilling this requirement. Other organizations might assign this responsibility to the health information director. In such a case, training staff in the management of information might be envisioned as a management of information process that needs to be planned and designed.

Q. Do we have to design and provide our own training? Or can we send staff to seminars or conferences off-site?
A. Either is fine. Your organization can choose to either provide

its own training or send staff off-site. The Joint Commission is concerned only that the training provided matches training needs. Therefore, even if you plan to send staff off-site for training, it would probably be useful to determine what your training needs are and then select training courses that fit those needs.

APPLICATION EXAMPLE 2.

Determining Training Needs for the Management of Information

To determine the training needs related to the management of information that exist in your organization, you might begin by defining the different job categories in your organization (for example, leaders, department or services directors, researchers, caregivers). Then, for each job category you might ask: What is this group's relationship to data and information? Do they generate data? Do they collect data? Do they organize it? Manipulate it? Do they make decisions based on it? The answers to these questions will help you understand the degree to which each group needs to be trained.

Different training programs can be designed or chosen based on the different needs. For example, department or service directors might attend a different course from unit nurses and other caregivers. In selecting or designing training programs, you might consider including instruction on the following:

- Understanding security and confidentiality of data and information;
- Using measurement instruments, statistical tools, and data analysis methods for transforming data into relevant information;
- Collecting unbiased data;
- Helping to interpret data;
- Using data and information in decision making;

- Supporting the participation of patients and family in care processes; and
- Using indicators to assess and improve systems and processes over time.

Transmission/Dissemination of Data (IM.5–IM.5.1)

RELATED STANDARDS

IM.5 (Capped at Score 2)

A 1 2 3 4 5 NA The transmission of data and information is timely and accurate.

IM.5.1 (Capped at Score 2)

A 1 2 3 4 5 NA The format and methods for disseminating data and information are standardized, whenever possible.

AN OVERVIEW OF REQUIREMENTS

Transmission refers to the sending of data and information from one location to another. Dissemination often occurs after data is transformed into information and refers to the distribution of information to different users. In the course of an average day, data and information is continually moving from one person or place to another, whether electronically or manually. The complexity of this activity ranges from ensuring that the emergency room physician has access to a patient's medical record to transmitting indicator reports to multiple external databases.

Organizations need to ensure that the integrity of data and information is maintained during transmission or dissemination and that these activities are carried out in a timely fashion. These processes should also provide for communication between the users and suppliers of data and information. For example, after the lab sends a report to a physician's office, a lab technologist should be available if the physician has any questions.

The format and methods used for transmitting and disseminating data and information should be based on the organization's and/or the users' needs and provide for easy retrievability. Whenever possible, data and information exchange formats should be standardized. For example, an organization should standardize its medical record format. On a smaller scale, the pharmacy might discourage the use of abbreviations or the use of the leading decimal point.

How Are These Standards Surveyed?

The surveyors will review any policies and procedures, meeting minutes, and other documents related to the transmission and dissemination of data and information. Surveyors will also ask leaders and staff about how well these processes are working. For example, they might ask clinical staff: How well does the design of the patient record meet your needs? Are results of diagnostic tests available in a timely fashion?

In addition, surveyors will observe how well these processes work as they review other standards in the *AMH*. For example, when reviewing the "Continuum of Care" standards, surveyors will observe how well information is transmitted and disseminated among various providers. This becomes particularly vital within a health care network. The whole intent of a network is to provide coordinated care among diverse health care providers. A major means for achieving the seamless coordination of care is a good information system that allows data and information to be shared, transmitted, and combined without interfering with or delaying patient care. When surveying a network, surveyors will pay careful attention to how well information is shared among providers.

Although the former medical records standards contained some requirements related to the medical record format, the 1995 standards are essentially new requirements. Therefore, in 1995, these standards are capped at a score of 2. This gives an organization a few years to come into full compliance with these standards. As part of the information needs assessment your organization conducts (IM.1), you should probably assess users' needs regarding transmission and dissemination of all types of data and information.

COMMON QUESTIONS

Q. What does the Joint Commission mean by "timely and accurate" transmission?
A. Essentially, the Joint Commission is concerned whether or not data and information is getting to users when it is needed and whether the integrity of this data and information is intact when it arrives. These are broad guidelines. Your organization will need to more specifically define "timely and accurate" transmission for the different types of data and information. For example, are radiology reports getting to the emergency room when needed? Are consultants' reports appearing in records soon enough to make continuing clinical decisions? Is information regarding changes in service (for example, radiology closing at 5 PM) made available?

As part of planning activities, you might ask users to relate what they consider to be timely transmission (for example, immediately? within one hour? within one day?) for different types of data and information (for example, the results of laboratory testing, articles they've requested from the library). You should also ask users whether the current formats and methods used for transmitting data and information are working well. Are users receiving complete information? Is the format in which the information is presented acceptable for their needs? For example, are data presented in a way that helps leaders make decisions?

Q. Besides patient care data, what are some examples of data and information in which timeliness and accuracy of transmission is a concern?
A. Data and information used in patient care activities will probably need to be transmitted in a more timely fashion than other types of data. However, organizations also participate in other activities that rely on the accurate and timely transmission of data and information. For example, when participating in an external database, an organization needs to keep up with the expectations for participation. When conducting clinical research, staff members depend on the accurate transmission of articles and literature. In addition, financial and employment data often need to be transmitted in a timely and accurate fashion.

Q. What does the Joint Commission mean by standardized exchange formats?
A. Just as organizations need to establish uniform data definitions (IM.3–IM.3.1) for the capture of data, they also need to consider standardizing the formats in which data and information are sent from one place to another. This applies to manual as well as computerized methods for transmitting data and information. Departments should probably have similar software so they can read each others' documents or have the capability to translate a document that is written in one computer program to another.

Organizations and departments that transmit information manually also run into language problems. For example, one department might use a different form than another department uses to report adverse drug events, and the pharmacy then must translate the different formats. A standardized form used by all departments would simplify this activity. Standardized exchange formats will also help facilitate communication between the supplier of data and information and the end user. Should the user need to determine the composition of the data (that is, where the numbers came from), a standardized report format would provide for such interface.

Data Integration/Linkages (IM.6–IM.6.3)

RELATED STANDARDS

IM.6 (Capped at Score 2)

A 1 2 3 4 5 NA The information-management function enables the combination of data and information; makes information from one system (clinical and/or organizational) available to another; provides reports; clarifies and interprets data and information; and enables linkage of patient care and non-patient care data and information over time among the organization's departments and provider resources for all care settings.

IM.6.1 (Capped at Score 3)

A 1 2 3 4 5 NA The retention time of medical record information is determined by law and regulation and by its use for patient care, legal, research, and/or educational purposes.

IM.6.2 (Capped at Score 2)

A 1 2 3 4 5 NA There are internal linkages among information-management processes related to important patient care and organizational functions described in this *Manual*.

IM.6.3 (Capped at Score 2)

A 1 2 3 4 5 NA The organization has access to external databases and bodies of expert health-related, administrative, and research knowledge, as required by its information-management needs.

AN OVERVIEW OF REQUIREMENTS

Before your organization can utilize and apply data, you must be able to compare the data across time, providers, departments, and so forth. Such comparisons allow organizations to analyze data trends, patterns, and variations to create a basis for decision making. To fully use data and information, your organization should have processes in place for the following:
- Gathering information from various sources;
- Providing and accessing longitudinal data and information;
- Using internal and external linkages, as needed;
- Analyzing situations based on this information; and
- Making decisions based on this analysis.

These standards place a heavy emphasis on establishing data linkages, which allow an organization to integrate different types of data (for example, clinical, financial, knowledge-based, external benchmarks). Most health care organizations currently have linkages in place to exchange information among patient care functions. However, the standards also require that organizations establish linkages among the organizational functions (for example, human resource and performance improvement) and between patient care and organizational functions (for example, clinical and financial).

These linkages provide staff with better access to the various types of data and information they need to carry out patient care, conduct research, and so forth. For example, some organizations are devising computerized systems that prompt physicians on the costs and effectiveness of various drugs at the bedside. By integrating cost and quality information, the physician is able to make a balanced decision about what drugs to order. Such linkages are also the basis for performance improvement. For example, the collection of organizationally determined performance indicators (including adverse events) can be used to assess and improve clinical, managerial, and support processes.

■ How Are These Standards Surveyed?

During the management of information meeting, surveyors will ask staff to describe the processes and mechanisms in place for integrating and linking data. They will be concerned about how these mechanisms ensure the linkage of data and information among the important functions identified in the *AMH*. The surveyors will also ask relevant questions as they meet with other staff and tour the building. For example, when visiting the library or resource center, the surveyor will be interested in the external linkages established to obtain knowledge-based information (see IM.9 for more on this).

Once again, because this is an organizational function, the organization's compliance with these standards will become evident during the course of the survey. For example, when assessing standards related to the "Leadership" chapter, surveyors might observe if administrative and financial systems are linked so that leaders have access to the data and information they need to make appropriate decisions.

Because IM.6, IM.6.2, and IM.6.3 are new standards, they are capped at a score of 2. This gives your organization some time to comply with these standards. As part of your information needs assessment, you should determine what linkages are most important to establish and then develop a plan for establishing those linkages over the next several years. Standard IM.6.1, which deals with the retention of the medical record, is not a new requirement. Organizations are expected to be in full compliance with this standard.

COMMON QUESTIONS

Q. What does the Joint Commission mean by linkages among functions?

A. Essentially, this means that data and information concerning any of the important functions identified in the *AMH* can be shared with appropriate data and information related to another function. For example, a social worker arranging for home care services (Continuum of Care) can locate information about that patient's nutritional care, if applicable (Care of Patients). Organizations should also be able to combine or integrate data and information related to different functions. For example, in making resource allocation decisions, an administrator may want to study how the number of registered nurses on a unit over time affected patient outcomes.

As part of the needs assessment, an organization might determine what type of information is currently being shared, and might be useful to share, among all the different functions. Then, it might assess how well the current processes for exchanging information are performing and develop priorities for improving and/or designing new linkages.

Q. What are some examples of data and information that can be combined?

A. The following are some examples of internal information systems that have potential for linkage:

- Clinical information systems (for example, medical record, pharmacy, laboratory systems);
- Systems for managing knowledge-based information (for example, interfaces between patient care data and clinical literature, and organizational data and management literature);
- Information systems for tracking, aggregating, and comparing internal information;
- Administrative and financial information systems (for example, billing);
- Instructional systems (for example, patient and family, staff);
- Research information systems; and
- Communication and office support systems (for example, word processing, electronic mail).

For example, clinical information might be linked to financial information to measure the effect of various practice patterns on costs of care. In addition, organizations should have access to external information systems (for example, comparative databases) and be able to combine this information with internal information as appropriate. These systems may be linked either manually or electronically.

Q. What would the Joint Commission consider "appropriate access" to external databases and bodies of knowledge-based resources?
A. Access to external databases or information resources should reflect your organization's information needs. As part of the needs assessment you conduct under IM.1, you should determine what users' needs are for external information. You should also consider any requirements for participating in external databases. (See the section on Comparative Information, IM.10, page 276, for more on this requirement.) In addition, your organization should have access to knowledge-based resources or the literature, which can be used for designing and redesigning processes and for problem-solving. (See the section on Knowledge-based Information, IM.9, page 265, for more on this requirement.)

Q. Does the Joint Commission expect us to have policies regarding the retention of all types of information or just of the medical record?
A. Standard IM.6.1 addresses only the retention of the medical record. The length of time the medical record should be retained will depend on the need to support patient care, performance improvement activities, organizational management, legal records, research, education, and the need to conform to applicable law and regulation.

However, one benefit of establishing data linkages is the ability to conduct longitudinal studies. Thus, organizations may also want to determine how long they want to retain other types of information including financial, demographic, patient satisfaction, and the like.

Patient-Specific Data and Information (IM.7–IM.7.10.1)

RELATED STANDARDS

IM.7 *The information management function provides for the definition, capture, analysis, transformation, transmission, and reporting of individual patient-specific data and information related to the process(es) and/or of outcome(s) of the patient's care.*

AN OVERVIEW OF REQUIREMENTS

Patient-specific information, which is commonly referred to as the medical record, is one of the four types of information your organization needs to manage. Your processes should provide for the use of patient-specific data and information to

- facilitate patient care;
- serve as a financial and legal record;
- aid in clinical research;
- support decision analysis; and
- provide a basis for professional and organizational performance improvement.

Your organization should be able to recall historical data about a specific patient as well as access data about current encounters.

Overall, these are not new standards; they formerly appeared in the "Medical Records" and "Medical Staff" chapters. Most organizations already have mechanisms in place designed to meet these requirements. However, organizations may want to reevaluate their current processes for managing patient-based information in light of the other standards in the "Management of Information" chapter.

Like Chapter 1, this chapter encourages organizations to view information as an important resource that must be managed across departments and functions. This means that the management of patient-based information should be tied to the management of other types of information. This is reflected in various standards throughout the chapter. For example, in establishing uniform data definitions (IM.3), organizations should ensure that the definitions used in the medical record are consistent with definitions used elsewhere, such as admissions or finance. In addition, to comply with IM.6, an organization needs to be able to link patient-based information with other types of information, such as financial or knowledge-based.

As part of the needs assessment in IM.1, your organization should consider whether the processes you currently have in place to manage patient-based information are sufficient. One part of this needs assessment is ensuring that your information processes are in line with your organization's mission and strategic plans. In light of the move toward managed or integrated care, your organization may want to consider redesigning current processes for managing patient-based information.

■ How Are These Standards Surveyed?

The surveyors will review your policies and procedures, medical staff rules and regulations, and any other documents related to the management of the medical record. The surveyors will then assess the quality of documentation and completeness of the medical record during open and closed record review. Since these are continuing requirements, organizations are expected to be in full compliance with these standards.

SPECIFIC REQUIREMENTS

Contents of the Medical Record (IM.7.1–IM.7.2.23)

IM.7.1 (No cap)

A 1 2 3 4 5 NA   The organization initiates and maintains a medical record for every individual assessed or treated. The medical record incorporates information from subsequent contacts between the patient and the organization.

IM.7.1.1 (Capped at Score 3)

A 1 2 3 4 5 NA   Entries in medical records are made only by individuals authorized to do so as specified in organization and medical staff policies.

IM.7.2 *The medical record contains sufficient information to identify the patient, support the diagnosis, justify the treatment, document the course and results accurately, and facilitate continuity of care among health care providers. Each medical record contains at least the following:*

IM.7.2.1 (Capped at Score 3)

A 1 2 3 4 5 NA   The patient's name, address, date of birth, and the name of any legally authorized representative;

IM.7.2.2 (Capped at Score 3)

A 1 2 3 4 5 NA   The patient's legal status, for patients receiving mental health services;

IM.7.2.3 (Capped at Score 3)

A 1 2 3 4 5 NA   Emergency care provided to the patient prior to arrival, if any;

IM.7.2.4 *The record and findings of the patient's assessment (see the "Assessment of Patients" chapter);*

> **IM.7.2.5 (Capped at Score 3)**
> B 1 2 3 4 5 NA   A statement of the conclusions or impressions drawn from the medical history and physical examination;
>
> **IM.7.2.6 (Capped at Score 3)**
> B 1 2 3 4 5 NA   The diagnosis or diagnostic impression;
>
> **IM.7.2.7 (Capped at Score 3)**
> B 1 2 3 4 5 NA   The reason(s) for admission or treatment;

IM.7.2.8 *The goals of treatment and the treatment plan;*

> **IM.7.2.9 (Capped at Score 3)**
> A 1 2 3 4 5 NA   Evidence of known advance directives;
>
> **IM.7.2.10 (Capped at Score 3)**
> A 1 2 3 4 5 NA   Evidence of informed consent for procedures and treatments for which informed consent is required by organizational policy;
>
> **IM.7.2.11 (Capped at Score 3)**
> A 1 2 3 4 5 NA   Diagnostic and therapeutic orders, if any;
>
> **IM.7.2.12 (Capped at Score 3)**
> A 1 2 3 4 5 NA   All diagnostic and therapeutic procedures and tests performed and the results;

IM.7.2.13 *All operative and other invasive procedures performed, using acceptable disease and operative terminology that includes etiology, as appropriate;*

IM.7.2.14 (Capped at Score 3)
A 1 2 3 4 5 NA   Progress notes made by the medical staff and other authorized individuals;

IM.7.2.15 (Capped at Score 3)
C 1 2 3 4 5 NA   All reassessments, when necessary;

IM.7.2.16 (Capped at Score 3)
C 1 2 3 4 5 NA   Clinical observations;

IM.7.2.17 (Capped at Score 3)
C 1 2 3 4 5 NA   The response to the care provided;

IM.7.2.18 (Capped at Score 3)
A 1 2 3 4 5 NA   Consultation reports;

IM.7.2.19 (Capped at Score 3)
A 1 2 3 4 5 NA   Every medication ordered or prescribed for an inpatient;

IM.7.2.20 (Capped at Score 3)
A 1 2 3 4 5 NA   Every dose of medication administered and any adverse drug reaction;

IM.7.2.21 (Capped at Score 3)
A 1 2 3 4 5 NA   Every medication dispersed to or prescribed for an ambulatory patient or an inpatient on discharge;

IM.7.2.22 (Capped at Score 3)
A 1 2 3 4 5 NA   All relevant diagnoses established during the course of care; and

IM.7.2.23 (Capped at Score 3)
A 1 2 3 4 5 NA   Any referrals and communications made to external or internal care providers and to community agencies.

To facilitate consistency and continuity in patient care, the Joint Commission requires that very specific data and information be included in all patient records (see Table 7, page 78). The record should contain sufficient information to identify the patient, support the diagnosis, justify the treatment, document the course of the treatment and its results accurately, and facilitate continuity of care among health care providers. Your organization can use the list in Table 7 as a basis for establishing what should be included in all medical records.

Discharge Information (IM.7.3–IM.7.3.2)

IM.7.3 (Capped at Score 3)

A 1 2 3 4 5 NA At discharge from inpatient care, a clinical resume concisely summarizes the reason for hospitalization, the significant findings, the procedures performed and treatment rendered, the patient's condition on discharge, and any specific instructions given to the patient and/or family, as pertinent.

IM.7.3.1 (Capped at Score 3)

A 1 2 3 4 5 NA A final progress note is substituted for the resume only for those patients with problems and interventions of a minor nature (as defined by the medical staff) who require less than a 48-hour period of hospitalization and in the case of normal newborn infants and uncomplicated obstetric deliveries.

IM.7.3.2 (Capped at Score 3)

A 1 2 3 4 5 NA A transfer summary may be substituted for the resume if the patient is transferred to a different level of hospitalization or residential care within the organization.

TABLE 7 Required Information for Hospital Medical Records

- The patient's name, address, date of birth, and the name of any legally authorized representative
- The patient's legal status, for patients receiving mental health services
- Emergency care provided, if any, to the patient prior to arrival
- The record and findings of the patient's assessment (see the "Assessment of Patients" chapter in the *AMH*)
- A statement of the conclusions or impressions drawn from the medical history and physical examination
- The diagnosis or diagnostic impression
- The reason(s) for admission or treatment
- The goals of treatment and the treatment plan
- Evidence of known advance directives
- Evidence of informed consent for procedures and treatments for which informed consent is required by organizational policy
- Diagnostic and therapeutic orders, if any
- All diagnostic and therapeutic procedures and tests performed and the results
- All operative and other invasive procedures performed, using acceptable disease and operative terminology that includes etiology, as appropriate
- Progress notes made by the medical staff and other authorized individuals
- All reassessments, when necessary
- Clinical observations
- The response to the care provided
- Consultation reports
- Every medication ordered or prescribed for an inpatient
- Every dose of medication administered and any adverse drug reaction
- Every medication dispersed to or prescribed for an ambulatory patient or an inpatient on discharge
- All relevant diagnoses established during the course of care
- Any referrals or communications made to external or internal care providers and to community agencies

Important information concerning a patient's care should be summarized and included in the medical record on discharge to facilitate continuity of care and communication among different providers. Typically, a clinical resume or discharge summary is included in the patient's record. The standards require that this discharge summary include the following:
- The reasons for hospitalization;
- The significant findings;
- The procedures performed and treatment rendered;
- The patient's condition on discharge; and
- Any specific instructions given to the patient and/or family, as pertinent.

Your organization may decide to require additional information in the summary. If so, your policies and procedures should reflect this.

In some circumstances, a lengthy discharge summary may be unnecessary. For example, a final progress note may be substituted for patients with problems and interventions of a minor nature who require less than a 48-hour period of hospitalization and in the case of normal newborn infants and uncomplicated obstetric deliveries. Your medical staff should define in writing the circumstances in which a final progress note is acceptable. You should also check your state's requirements regarding this.

A transfer summary may also be substituted for a clinical resume when a patient is transferred from one level of care (for example, hospital) to another level of care (for example, residential or partial hospitalization) within the same organization such that the caregivers change. If the caregivers remain the same, a progress note may be sufficient. However, if a patient is discharged to ambulatory (outpatient) care, the medical record should include a clinical resume that summarizes the previous levels of care. Again, your organization's policies for when a transfer summary is acceptable should be documented.

Operative or Other Invasive Procedures (IM.7.4–IM.7.4.3.6)

IM.7.4 *The medical record of patients undergoing operative or other invasive procedures and/or anesthesia includes the additional following information:*

IM.7.4.1 (Capped at Score 3)

A 1 2 3 4 5 NA   The licensed independent practitioner who is responsible for the patient records a preoperative diagnosis prior to surgery.

IM.7.4.2 (Capped at Score 3)

A 1 2 3 4 5 NA   Operative reports are dictated or written in the medical record immediately after surgery and describe the findings, the technical procedures used, the specimen(s) removed, the postoperative diagnosis, and the name of the primary surgeon and any assistants.

IM.7.4.2.1 (Capped at Score 3)

A 1 2 3 4 5 NA   The completed operative report is authenticated by the surgeon and filed in the medical record as soon as possible after surgery.

IM.7.4.2.2 (Capped at Score 3)

A 1 2 3 4 5 NA   When the operative report is not placed in the medical record immediately after surgery (for example, there is a transcription and/or filing delay), an operative progress note is entered in the medical record immediately after surgery to provide pertinent information for any individual required to attend to the patient.

IM.7.4.3 *Postoperative documentation includes at least a record of*

IM.7.4.3.1 *vital signs and level of consciousness;*

IM.7.4.3.2 *medications (including intravenous fluids) and blood and blood components;*

IM.7.4.3.3 *any unusual events or postoperative complications, including blood transfusion reactions, and the management of those events;*

IM.7.4.3.4 (Capped at Score 3)
A 1 2 3 4 5 NA identification of who provided direct patient care nursing services and who supervised that care if it was provided by someone other than a qualified registered nurse;

IM.7.4.3.5 *the patient's discharge from the postanesthesia care area by the responsible licensed independent practitioner or by the use of relevant discharge criteria; and*

IM.7.4.3.5.1 (Capped at Score 4)
A 1 2 3 4 5 NA The criteria are approved by the medical staff and rigorously applied to determine the patient's readiness for discharge.

IM.7.4.3.6 (Capped at Score 3)
A 1 2 3 4 5 NA the name of the licensed independent practitioner responsible for the discharge.

In addition to the specific information outlined in Table 7, the surgical record should document all aspects of a surgical patient's preoperative, operative, and postoperative events, including the following:
- The preoperative diagnosis;
- A complete description of the surgical procedure and findings;
- The identity of all practitioners involved in the process;

- The postoperative course; and
- Evidence of the patient's readiness for discharge from the postanesthesia care area and the discharge.

Operative reports should be thoroughly and consistently recorded in the medical record in accordance with organizational policies and procedures and applicable state laws. This requirement applies to all outpatients and inpatients, including donors and recipients of organs and tissues.

Ambulatory Patients (IM.7.5–IM.7.5.1)

IM.7.5 (Capped at Score 4)

A 1 2 3 4 5 NA The medical record for patients receiving continuing ambulatory care services includes a list of known significant diagnoses, conditions, procedures, drug allergies, and medications.

IM.7.5.1 (Capped at Score 4)

A 1 2 3 4 5 NA The list is initiated and maintained for each patient by the third visit.

To promote continuity of care among providers or for a single provider over time, records are maintained for patients receiving ambulatory care services. When patients receive continuing ambulatory care (that is, three or more visits), a summary list is included in the record that contains the following:
- Known significant medical diagnoses and conditions;
- Known significant surgical and invasive procedures;
- Known adverse and allergic drug reactions; and
- Medications known to be prescribed for and/or used by the patient.

Known refers to information gathered as part of the ambulatory care assessment and treatment. If a patient is seen in more than one clinic and if each clinic maintains a separate medical record, the records should indicate, at a minimum, when information is contained in another record or another section of the medical record.

Emergency Care (IM.7.6–IM.7.6.2)

IM.7.6 *When emergency care is provided,*

IM.7.6.1 *the following additional information is required in the medical record:*

IM.7.6.1.1 (Capped at Score 3)
A 1 2 3 4 5 NA Time and means of arrival;

IM.7.6.1.2 (Capped at Score 3)
A 1 2 3 4 5 NA The patient's leaving against medical advice; and

IM.7.6.1.3 (Capped at Score 3)
A 1 2 3 4 5 NA Conclusions at termination of treatment, including final disposition, condition at discharge, and instructions for follow-up care.

IM.7.6.2 (Capped at Score 3)
A 1 2 3 4 5 NA When authorized by the patient or his or her legally authorized representative, a copy of the record of emergency services provided is available to the practitioner or medical organization responsible for follow-up care.

The medical records of patients who have received emergency care should contain additional information, including
- Time and means of arrival;
- The patient's leaving against medical advice, if applicable; and
- Conclusions at termination of treatment, including final disposition, patient's condition at discharge, and any instruction for follow-up care. Organizations should ensure that a copy of the record of emergency services is provided to the practitioner or organization responsible for the patient's follow-up care.

Timely Completion of Record (IM.7.7–IM.7.7.2)

IM.7.7 *Medical record data and information are managed in a timely manner.*

IM.7.7.1 (Capped at Score 4)

A 1 2 3 4 5 NA All significant clinical information pertaining to the patient is entered into the medical record as soon as possible after its occurrence.

IM.7.7.2 (No Cap)

A 1 2 3 4 5 NA Medical records of discharged patients must be completed within a time period specified in the medical staff rules and regulations, not to exceed 30 days.

Practitioners need to complete entries in a timely manner if that clinical information is to be valuable in the concurrent and ongoing care of a patient. Documentation of patient medical history, physical examination, and operative reports is particularly important but not more or less important than other documentation. For the most part, it is up to the organization to determine the specific time frames for entries to be made. These time frames should be documented in policies and procedures. However, the standards do require some time frames:

1. All inpatient records reflect that all assessments and screenings including medical history, physical examination, and nursing assessment are completed on each patient within 24 hours of admission (PE.1.7.1). This time frame applies for weekend, holiday, and week-day admissions. A medical history and physical assessment must be completed or thoroughly updated within 30 days prior to admission. If significant changes occur between the time of documentation and hospital admission, they are recorded at the time of admission. If a patient is readmitted for treatment of the same or a related problem within 30 days following discharge from the hospital, an interval history and physical examination report reflecting any subsequent changes may be used in the medical record, provided that the original information is included in the record.
2. Operative reports must be completed "immediately" after surgery.
3. When an autopsy is performed, provisional anatomic diagnoses are recorded in the medical record within three days, and the complete protocol is included in the record within 60 days, unless the medical staff establishes exceptions for special studies.

At discharge, a complete medical record is important; however, the time frame is less critical. The Joint Commission requires that all records be completed within 30 days after discharge. A medical record is considered complete when (1) its contents reflect the diagnosis, diagnostic test results, therapy, patient's condition, in-hospital progress, and patient's condition at discharge; and (2) its contents, including any required clinical resume or final progress notes, are assembled and authenticated, and all final diagnoses and any complications are recorded without the use of symbols or abbreviations.

Verbal Orders (IM.7.8–IM.7.8.2.1)

IM.7.8 (Capped at Score 3)

A 1 2 3 4 5 NA Verbal orders of authorized individuals are accepted and transcribed by qualified personnel who are identified by title or category in the medical staff rules and regulations.

IM.7.8.1 (Capped at Score 3)

A 1 2 3 4 5 NA Verbal orders for medications are accepted only by personnel so designated in the medical staff rules and regulations and are authenticated by the prescribing practitioner within the stated period of time.

IM.7.8.2 (Capped at Score 2)

A 1 2 3 4 5 NA The medical staff defines any category of diagnostic or therapeutic verbal orders associated with any potential hazard to the patient.

IM.7.8.2.1 (Capped at Score 3)

A 1 2 3 4 5 NA Such verbal orders are authenticated by the practitioner responsible for the patient within a time frame defined in the medical staff rules and regulations.

Because verbal orders can adversely affect patient care quality, an organization needs to design a mechanism for receiving, transcribing, and authenticating verbal orders. In their rules and regulations, the medical staff needs to establish the following:
- Which qualified personnel are allowed to take verbal orders (for example, nurses, pharmacists);
- How to handle verbal orders regarding medications;
- What verbal orders might be associated with a potential

hazard to patients and how to handle those orders; and
- Within what time frame do verbal orders need to be authenticated (for example, within 24 hours).

When establishing a time frame for authentication, applicable state law should be considered.

Authentication of Entries (IM.7.9–IM.7.9.3)

IM.7.9 (Capped at Score 3)
A 1 2 3 4 5 NA All entries in the medical records are dated and authenticated, and a method is established to identify the authors of entries.

IM.7.9.1 (Capped at Score 2)
A 1 2 3 4 5 NA Authentication may be by written signatures or initials, rubber-stamp signatures, or computer key.

IM.7.9.2 (Capped at Score 3)
A 1 2 3 4 5 NA When rubber-stamp signatures or computer key are authorized, the individual whose signature the stamp represents or whose computer key is authorized signs a statement that he or she alone will use the stamp or the code for the computer key. This statement is filed in the organization's administrative offices.

IM.7.9.2.1 (Capped at Score 4)
A 1 2 3 4 5 NA Such a stamp or code for the computer key is not used by another individual.

IM.7.9.3 (Capped at Score 3)
A 1 2 3 4 5 NA The appropriate practitioner authenticates the parts of the medical record for which he or she is responsible.

Making entries in the medical record is a privilege. Thus, your organization should have a system in place that limits access to the medical records to those personnel authorized to make entries. To maintain the security of this system, all authors need to authenticate that their entries are accurate (for example, by signing the entry). Any entries in the medical records by house staff or nonphysicians that require countersigning by supervisory or attending medical staff members are defined in the medical staff rules and regulations. Countersignature is one form of evidence of supervision.

Divergent Record Components (IM.7.10–IM.7.10.1)

IM.7.10 (Capped at Score 3)

A 1 2 3 4 5 NA   When a patient is admitted to the hospital or appears for a prescheduled ambulatory care appointment, the organization uses a patient information system to routinely assemble all divergently located record components. The system also ensures that all record components are assembled in a timely manner, as needed for patients seen for unscheduled ambulatory and emergency services visits.

IM.7.10.1 (Capped at Score 3)

A 1 2 3 4 5 NA   The medical record or computer system indicates when a portion of the record has been filed elsewhere to alert authorized personnel of the portion's existence.

Practitioners have on hand or have ready access to any relevant information about any care the patient may have previously received anywhere in the organization, including its ambulatory or emergency service. This applies if the patient is admitted to the hospital or is being seen for a prescheduled ambulatory care visit as well as for an unscheduled outpatient visit or an emergency service visit. Such information facilitates continuity of care among multiple providers and over time for a single provider. This information is provided in a timely manner by hard copy or screen display.

COMMON QUESTIONS

Q. How should verbal orders be documented in the medical record?
A. A verbal order may be transcribed in the medical record by a qualified staff person, as defined by medical staff rules and regulations. However, this entry needs to be authenticated by the practitioner who issued the order. The time frame in which verbal orders should be authenticated should also be defined in the medical staff rules and regulations and comply with any regulations or laws.

Q. Why is authentication of all entries required?
A. Authentication means that the author is identified and the entry is complete and accurately reflects the intention of the author. Authentication is not an issue when a practitioner physically signs an entry that has just been made. However, entries are often given over the phone or by transcription. In such instances, the transcriptionist cannot sign the name of the person who dictated the entry; rather, the transcriptionist can only identify the author of the entry. An authentication is not complete until the author validates the content of the transcribed entry.

Q. Which methods of authentication are acceptable? Which are not?
A. The process of authentication must provide a practitioner with the opportunity to read his or her entry and validate what

it says. When a practitioner physically signs an entry, the Joint Commission presumes he or she has read it. The Joint Commission applies this same principle when authentication is handled electronically.

There are some systems that enable a practitioner to dictate an entry and then key in a code that will electronically affix a signature to that entry when it is transcribed. Such a system does not meet the intent of the standards because it does not provide an opportunity for the practitioner to proofread and validate the content. However, the Joint Commission will accept a system that provides practitioners with an opportunity to review a transcription of their entry before entering a key code that affixes their electronic signature.

Only the practitioner should be able to use his or her electronic code. The same applies with manual tools, such as rubber stamps. Only the practitioner should be able to use his or her rubber stamp. The standards require that practitioners sign a document that says something to the effect of, "I will keep the stamp in my possession, and I am the only one who can use it."

"Blanket authentication" is another method that fails to meet the intent of the standard. Practitioners cannot sign a form (for example, on the front of the chart), that says something to the effect of "By signing this form, I hereby authenticate all my entries in this record." Again, practitioners must authenticate each entry.

Aggregate Data/Information (IM.8–IM.8.1.12)

RELATED STANDARDS

IM.8 (Capped at Score 2)

A 1 2 3 4 5 NA   The information-management function provides for the definition, capture, analysis, transmission, and reporting of data and information that can be aggregated to support managerial decisions and operations, performance-improvement activities, and patient care.

AN OVERVIEW OF REQUIREMENTS

The Joint Commission defines "aggregate" as the "combination of standardized data and information." Thus, this standard is intrinsically tied to standard IM.6, which requires organizations to have processes in place that allow for different types of data and information to be integrated and linked. IM.6 asks whether your organization has the necessary processes in place to link various types of data. IM.8 asks whether you are capable of combining various types of data and information over time. The standards under IM.8 also ask whether these data are being used by leaders and staff. It is not enough to simply establish mechanisms that enable your organization to create aggregate data. Surveyors will want to know if leaders and staff use aggregate data in making managerial decisions, in performance-improvement activities, and in patient care.

By assessing data and information over time or making internal or external comparisons, staff can determine patterns in performance. For example, organizational leaders can track patient satisfaction over time and across units to identify trends. Leaders might go on to compare patient satisfaction against clinical outcomes. The organization can also use aggregate data to make external comparisons, which is required under IM.10. For example, staff can compare aggregate outcome data (such as, for CABG procedures) to outcomes at another organization(s) as a way of identifying opportunities for improvement. Other examples of patient data that may be aggregated are data for blood usage review, operative and invasive procedure review, and medication usage evaluation to improve performance.

As part of its information needs assessment (IM.1), your organization should assess users' needs and different uses for aggregate data and information. The standards under IM.8 require that you aggregate and analyze certain types of data and information (for example, data and information related to the safety of the environment). These requirements are discussed in more detail in the pages that follow.

■ How Are These Standards Surveyed?

The surveyors will review any documents (for example, a management of information plan, policies and procedures, meeting minutes, and so forth) and speak with staff to determine if you assessed and planned for your organization's needs for aggregate data and information. In addition, when visiting particular areas or talking to various staff members, the surveyors will ask staff members to describe the types of aggregate data that are available to them to support decision making, operations, improvement activities, and patient care activities.

Some of these standards are capped at a score of 2. Those that are not capped are typically continuing requirements (for example, aggregation of pharmacy transactions). Organizations should already have mechanisms in place to meet these requirements. For newer requirements, your organization should plan how it intends to meet these requirements within the next several years.

SPECIFIC REQUIREMENTS

Safety and Environment Hazards (IM.8.1.1–IM.8.1.3)

IM.8.1 *Data and information that can be aggregated include at least the following:*

IM.8.1.1 (Capped at Score 3)
A 1 2 3 4 5 NA   Pharmacy transactions as required by applicable law and as necessary to adequately control and account for all drugs, including:

IM.8.1.1.1 (Capped at Score 3)
A 1 2 3 4 5 NA   Maintaining a means of identifying the signatures of all practitioners authorized to prescribe/order medications; and

IM.8.1.1.2 (Capped at Score 3)
A 1 2 3 4 5 NA   A listing of practitioners' Drug Enforcement Administration numbers, where required.

IM.8.1.2 *Information about hazards and safety practices used to identify safety management issues to be addressed by the safety committee, including:*

IM.8.1.2.1 (Capped at Score 3)
A 1 2 3 4 5 NA   Summaries of the deficiencies, problems, failures, and user errors in safety management, life safety management, equipment management, and utilities management, as well as relevant published reports of hazards associated with any of these areas;

IM.8.1.2.2 (Capped at Score 3)
A 1 2 3 4 5 NA   Documented surveys, at least semiannually, of all areas of the facility to identify environmental hazards and unsafe practices; and

IM.8.1.2.3 (Capped at Score 3)
A 1 2 3 4 5 NA   Reports and investigations of all incidents involving property damage, occupational illness, or patient, personnel, or visitor injury.

IM.8.1.3 (Capped at Score 3)

A 1 2 3 4 5 NA Records of radionuclides and radiopharmaceuticals, including the radionuclide's identity, the date received, method of receipt, activity, recipient's identity, date administered, and disposal;

With the Joint Commission's new emphasis on performance, many standards in the *AMH* encourage organizations to design effective processes and systems so that "things are done right the first time." However, given the nature of health care, organizations are still required to monitor or establish controls when a risk to the patient is great. These standards require your organization to track the following:

- Pharmacy transactions as required by applicable law and as necessary to adequately control and account for all drugs;
- Information about hazards and safety practices to identify safety management issues; and
- Records of radionuclides and radiopharmaceuticals.

To adequately detect trends and patterns in these areas, data need to be aggregated over time. These aggregate data should be used by organizations to take appropriate actions when necessary. For example, the safety committee should continuously review aggregate information related to environmental hazards and unsafe practices (for example, patient falls, drug poisoning). When a special cause is detected, staff should immediately investigate the cause and take corrective action.

Meeting External Regulatory Requirements (IM.8.1.4)

IM.8.1.4 (Capped at Score 3)

A 1 2 3 4 5 NA Records of any required reporting to proper authorities;

As part of its needs assessment, your organization should inventory the different data and information you are collecting and aggregating to meet external regulatory requirements (for example, sending infection data to the Centers for Disease Control or cancer data to the American Cancer Society's cancer registry). The following are some examples of data and information that your organization may be tracking for reporting purposes:
- Birth and death registration;
- Transfusion-related fatalities;
- Contagious diseases;
- Adverse drug reactions;
- Immunizations;
- Abuse victims;
- Gunshot wounds;
- Reports to the FDA and/or the manufacturer of a medical-device-related death or serious injury or illness caused or contributed to by that device; and
- Any required records for adequate control and accountability for medical devices. Organizations will probably already have mechanisms in place to meet this requirement. However, as part of your organization's planning activities, you may want to check if any duplicate reporting efforts are going on. You should also consider how leaders and staff can use these aggregate data in making managerial decisions and operations, performance-improvement, or patient care processes.

Coding and Retrieval Systems (IM.8.1.5–IM.8.1.7)

IM.8.1.5 (Capped at Score 3)
A 1 2 3 4 5 NA   A coding and retrieval system for medical records by diagnosis and procedure;

IM.8.1.6 (Capped at Score 3)
A 1 2 3 4 5 NA A coding and retrieval system for patient demographic information;

IM.8.1.6.1 (Capped at Score 3)
A 1 2 3 4 5 NA A continuously maintained control register for emergency and outpatient services includes at least the following information for every individual seeking care: identification, such as name, age, and sex; date, time, and means of arrival; nature of complaint; disposition; and time of departure.

IM.8.1.7 (Capped at Score 3)
A 1 2 3 4 5 NA A coding and retrieval system for financial information;

Most organizations already have systems in place that enable the retrieval of aggregate data and information from the medical record according to diagnosis. However, the standards also require that your organization develop systems that enable the retrieval of patient demographic and financial data and information. Again, these standards emphasize the use of these data in managerial decisions and operations, performance improvement processes, and patient care. These systems should enable your organization to continually assess different aspects of performance or to carry out special studies.

Performance Monitoring and Improvement (IM.8.1.8–IM.8.1.9)

IM.8.1.8 (No cap)
A 1 2 3 4 5 NA Measures (that is, indicators) of processes and outcomes for assessing performance;

IM.8.1.9 (Capped at Score 4)

A 1 2 3 4 5 NA   Summaries of actions taken as the result of organizationwide performance-improvement activities, including risk management, utilization review, infection control, and safety management;

The improving organizational performance standards require organizations to continuously measure and assess various aspects of their performance. Organizations need to continuously assess various process and outcome measures and use these findings in setting priorities for improvement. Thus, as part of your organization's information-planning activities, it needs to assess what aggregate data and information needs to be captured to fulfill these requirements.

Performance-improvement activities are often occurring simultaneously throughout an organization. For example, a hospital might be redesigning its admitting process while an emergency room is improving its waiting time. At the same time, an organization must continue to carry out risk management, utilization review, infection control, and safety management activities. To keep track of all these activities and ensure that they are coordinated, organizations should track any actions taken.

Practitioner Credentialing (IM.8.1.10)

IM.8.1.10 (Capped at Score 3)

A 1 2 3 4 5 NA   Practitioner-specific information for licensed independent practitioners, as defined in the "Medical Staff" chapter of the *AMH*;

As part of credentialing and appointment or reappointment activities, organizations need to track aggregate data and information about the licensed independent practitioners on staff. Organizations have always been required to capture these data under the medical staff requirements. As part of your information-planning activities, your organization might assess whether these data, when aggregated, are being used in additional ways (for example, to identify educational and improvement opportunities).

Operational Decision Making and Clinical Research (IM.8.1.11–IM.8.1.12)

IM.8.1.11 (Capped at Score 3)
A 1 2 3 4 5 NA The ability to gather accurate, timely information for both operational decision making and planning purposes; and

IM.8.1.12 (Capped at Score 2)
A 1 2 3 4 5 NA Data and information to support clinical research, as desired.

These two standards encourage your organization to assess what aggregate data and information are needed to support clinical research and decision-making activities. This should be done as part of your organization's information-planning activities. Your organization may have specific needs for aggregate data in addition to the different types of aggregate data and information identified under IM.8. For example, organizational leaders might want to track costs, outcomes, patient satisfaction, and other measures related to a high-volume procedure (for example, congestive heart failure or myocardial infarction). Or clinical leaders may want to conduct research related to total hip replacement. They may want to aggregate data from patients requiring a total hip replacement and analyze the results of various treatment options to determine efficacy.

COMMON QUESTIONS

Q. Will surveyors check if all the different types of data listed under IM.8 are in our information system?
A. Surveyors will ask what types of data and information are aggregated in your organization. They may ask to see some examples of aggregate data, particularly related to requirements under Standard IM.8. This sampling is typical of the Joint Commission's survey process. There is generally not enough time to review every piece of data and information in your organization.

Q. Do coding and retrieval systems (for example, for patient demographic and financial information) need to cover outpatient and ambulatory care?
A. Yes. As described under Standard IM.6, you should have data linkages among your organization's departments and provider resources for all care settings.

Q. Will organizations that use a lot of aggregate data and information do better on a survey?
A. Not necessarily. The point of these standards is not to encourage organizations to obtain more data. Some organizations already suffer an overabundance of data—a syndrome known as DRIP or "Data Rich, Information Poor." The point of these standards is to ensure that your internal and external users have the data and information they need to carry out patient care, make managerial decisions, conduct research, and continuously improve performance. The amount of aggregate data and information captured will depend on your organization's mission, scope of care, and available resources.

Knowledge-based Data/Information (IM.9–IM.9.6)

RELATED STANDARDS

IM.9 *The management of knowledge-based information (also referred to as "literature") provides for the identification, organization, retrieval, analysis, delivery, and reporting of clinical and managerial journal literature, reference information, and research data for use in designing, managing, and improving patient-specific and organizational processes.*

Knowledge-based data and information, or what is traditionally referred to as "literature," consists of systems, resources, and services that provide leaders and staff with authoritative and up-to-date print and nonprint information resources. Knowledge-based data and information is essential in helping health professionals acquire and maintain the knowledge and skills they need to care for patients, support clinical and managerial decision making, and provide needed information and education to patients and families.

Your organization's library and information services should meet the following demands:
- Respond to information requests from the clinical and management staff, other organizational staff, and patients and their families, as appropriate;
- Provide information in advance by anticipating information needs and systematically linking the literature with clinical and organizational processes; and
- Provide relevant, current, and accurate information within appropriate time frames and in formats appropriate to recipients' needs.

For the most part, these standards appeared in the 1993 "Medical Library" chapter. Organizations will typically already have mechanisms in place to meet these requirements. However, as with other types of data and information, organizations should reevaluate their current processes for managing knowledge-based information in light of the other standards in the "Management of Information" chapter. As part of the needs assessment under IM.1, your organization should consider whether the processes you currently have in place are sufficient.

In particular, you should assess your organization's ability to link with other internal information systems and with appropriate external databases and information networks (IM.6, IM.9.2.1.2, IM.9.2.1.3). For example, can you interface patient care data and clinical literature? Also, can you obtain information resources not owned by the organization (for example, through reciprocal sharing agreements)?

■ How Are These Standards Surveyed?

The surveyors will review any documents (for example, written plans, needs surveys, notes, or meeting minutes) related to your organization's assessment of knowledge-based information needs. Surveyors will ask users if they have access to knowledge-based information when they need it. For example, in visits to patient care settings, surveyors may ask caregivers if they have ready access to clinical, scientific, and managerial information. Finally, the surveyor will visit the resource center(s) and ask the director to describe the organization's planning activities for knowledge-based information. (Chapter 3, page 123, provides more details on the visit to the resource center).

The only standards under IM.9 that are capped at a score of 2 are IM.9.2.1.2 through IM.9.2.1.3. Both are related to information linkages. Besides these, organizations are expected to be in full compliance with the standards under IM.9.

Planning (IM.9.1–IM.9.2.1.3)

IM.9.1 (Capped at Score 3)

A 1 2 3 4 5 NA   The organization provides systems, resources, and services to meet its informational, educational, and, when appropriate, research-related needs for knowledge-based information and literature.

IM.9.2 (Capped at Score 3)

A 1 2 3 4 5 NA   The extent of knowledge-based information services, resources, and systems (for example, professional library and health information services) is related not only to the organizational services provided, but also to the needs of the medical and nursing staffs, administrators and managers, other health professional staff, other organization staff, students, patients and their families, and researchers.

IM.9.2.1 *The assessment of organizational needs for knowledge-based information considers*

IM.9.2.1.1 (Capped at Score 3)

A 1 2 3 4 5 NA   the need for accessibility and timeliness;

IM.9.2.1.2 (Capped at Score 2)

A 1 2 3 4 5 NA   the need to link with the organization's internal information systems; and

IM.9.2.1.3 (Capped at Score 2)

A 1 2 3 4 5 NA   the need to link with appropriate external databases and information networks.

These standards require that your organization assess its current needs for knowledge-based resources and plan accordingly. As part of this needs assessment, you should consider the following:

- *The need for accessibility.* For example, do physicians have access to medical knowledge databases? Are caregivers familiar with various types of information technology that allow them to access and manage medical information for patient care?
- *The need for timeliness.* For example, when conducting clinical research, can staff obtain requested literature within a day or two?
- *The need to link with the organization's internal information systems.* For example, when making clinical decisions, can caregivers access the clinical literature?
- *The need to link with appropriate external databases and information networks.* For example, can your organization obtain resources either on-line or through contractual agreements with other libraries?

Systems in Place (IM.9.3–IM.9.6)

IM.9.3 (Capped at Score 3)

A 1 2 3 4 5 NA Systems and structures (electronic or paper based) provide for the appropriate identification, organization, retrieval, analysis, delivery, and reporting of knowledge-based information and literature to meet identified needs.

IM.9.4 (Capped at Score 3)

A 1 2 3 4 5 NA Accessible knowledge-based information resources include clinical and management literature (in appropriate formats, including paper or electronic journals, books, technical reports, and audiovisuals); externally produced databases; practice guidelines; and information in multiple formats for patient education (brochures, articles, pamphlets, audiovisual materials, and models).

IM.9.4.1 (Capped at Score 3)
A 1 2 3 4 5 NA The organization's knowledge-based information resources are authoritative and up to date.

IM.9.5 (Capped at Score 3)
A 1 2 3 4 5 NA The pharmacy, medical, and nursing staff has access to poison-control information.

IM.9.6 (Capped at Score 3)
A 1 2 3 4 5 NA A hospital formulary or drug list is readily available to the staff who use it.

For knowledge-based resources to be accessible to everyone who needs them, your organization must have the following systems in place (either electronic or paper based):

- *Systems to manage the resources currently available in the organization.* For example, automated or paper catalogs with access by author, title, journal, and subject and/or providing location of information and other lists of resources. Such systems and structures allow your organization to organize, locate, use, and share information and resources that are currently available.
- *Systems for identifying resources.* Examples of electronic or paper-based systems that facilitate the identification of knowledge-based information include subject indexes (for example, Index Medicus, Medline) and systems that provide access to medical and university libraries at the international, national, regional, and local levels.

- *Systems for locating and delivering appropriate resources.* These include networks that provide access to other library holdings, clearinghouses, commercial information services, and international, national, regional, and local systems for sharing resources (for example, the British Library, the National Library of Medicine and its National Network of Libraries of Medicine, local consortia).
- *Systems and structures that provide appropriate controls to assure uniformity, completeness, and compatibility with bibliographic and other records.* Examples include subject thesauri (for example, Medical Subject Headings); classification systems (the National Library of Medicine Classification System); the MARC format for bibliographic description; agreements, regulations, policies and procedures for cooperative resource sharing; and codes for interlibrary lending (for example, the ILL code of the American Library Association).

These standards also require that poison-control and formulary information be readily available to staff. A poison-control center hotline is usually the most effective, up-to-date source of information.

COMMON QUESTIONS

Q. Should this needs assessment be separate from the assessment of information needs required under IM.1.1? How is the assessment of knowledge-based needs supposed to be documented?

A. An organization is supposed to assess users' needs for all types of information, including knowledge-based information. An organization might choose to assess needs for knowledge-based information at the same time it assesses needs for other types of data and information. However, on a practical level, this might be difficult. Instead, management of information plans might assign the assessment of these needs to the resource center or librarian. Figure 5, page 107, provides a survey your organization might use to assess knowledge-based needs. In such instances, the needs assessment might be documented in a separate plan, meeting minutes, a survey of needs, or elsewhere.

Q. What if an organization is small? Do we need our own library?
A. The Joint Commission is concerned that staff have access to literature. Information is accessible in one or more of the following ways: immediately at the work site; within the hospital in a shared central collection (for example, a professional library); and/or from outside sources with acceptable time delays (for example, from vendors or other institutions).

Q. What authoritative resources does the Joint Commission recognize?
A. We do not require you to have access to any specific resources. Rather, we are concerned that the resources you access and use are respected and provide authoritative and up-to-date scientific, clinical, and managerial knowledge. Examples of authoritative resources include reference materials, such as *Selected List of Books and Journals for the Small Medical Library* (referred to as the Brandon-Hill list), which is published every other year by the Medical Library Association (MLA) in the *Bulletin of the MLA,* and the *Library for Internists,* published by the American College of Physicians every three years in the Annals of Internal Medicine. Other methods of selecting authoritative, up-to-date resources include scanning databases and publishing information, following customer recommendations, and using reviews.

FIGURE 5 User Survey for Knowledge-Based Information—Provided by New Jersey Medical Libraries

I.D. Number_____

PLEASE PRINT LEGIBLY AND ANSWER ALL QUESTIONS.
Your answers are confidential.

General Questions

1. What is your current status? (Check one.)
   a. Resident ....( )
   b. Physician post residency ....( )

2. On average, during the past 12 months, how frequently have you come in contact with this library, by personal visit, mail or telephone, or indirectly by having someone else contact the library on your behalf? (Check one answer.)
   a. Daily ....( )
   b. At least once a week ....( )
   c. At least once a month ....( )
   d. At least once during the year ....( )
   e. Not at all during last 12 months ....( )

3. Indicate materials or services used from the library during the past twelve months. (Check all that apply.)
   a. Journal(s) or newspaper(s) and/or audiovisuals ....( )
   b. Books ....( )
   c. Equipment or computer software ....( )
   d. Reference Service(s) ....( )
   e. Interlibrary Loan Service ....( )
   f. Card catalog and/or indexes ....( )
   g Computerized literature search performed by library staff .....( )
   h. Used library computer to do my own on-line searches ....( )
   i. Photocopy service ....( )
   j. Telefacsimile ....( )
   k. Other ....( )
   l. Nothing ....( )

Clinical Decision-Making Questions

4. What is the principal diagnosis of the patient to which your request to the librarian is related?

Continued on next page

An example of a survey that an organization might use to assess knowledge-based needs.

FIGURE 5 User Survey for Knowledge-Based Information— Provided by New Jersey Medical Libraries *(continued)*

5. How would you characterize the *clinical* value of the information you received from the librarian in response to your request? (Check one answer for each statement.)

	Yes	No
a. Most of it was irrelevant	( )	( )
b. Refreshed my memory of details of facts	( )	( )
c. It did (or will) contribute to higher quality care	( )	( )
d. Obtained new information	( )	( )
e. Found little or nothing of clinical value	( )	( )
f. Substantiated what I already knew or suspected	( )	( )
g. Overall was inaccurate or out of date	( )	( )
h. It did (or will) contribute to better informed clinical decisions	( )	( )
i. None of the above	( )	( )
j. Other (please specify)_____	( )	( )

6. As a result of this clinically oriented information received from the librarian, did you (or will you) handle any aspect of the patient's care *differently* than you would have handled it otherwise? (Check one answer.)
   a. Definitely yes .... ( )
   b. Probably yes .... ( )
   c. Probably not .... ( )
   d. Definitely not .... ( )

7. If you answered definitely yes or probably yes, please assess the importance of the change(s) for the optimal care of the patient. (Circle the number.)

   UNIMPORTANT 1 ... 2 ... 3 ... 4 ... 5 IMPORTANT

8. Did this information provided by the librarian change (or will change) any of the following? (Check one answer for each item.)

	Yes	No	Unknown	Not Applicable
a. Diagnosis	( )	( )	( )	( )
b. Diagnostic tests	( )	( )	( )	( )
c. Drug treatment	( )	( )	( )	( )
d. Choice of other treatment	( )	( )	( )	( )
e. Length of hospital stay				
(increase)	( )	( )	( )	( )
(decrease)	( )	( )	( )	( )
f. Posthospital care or treatment	( )	( )	( )	( )
g. Advice given to patient	( )	( )	( )	( )

FIGURE 5 User Survey for Knowledge-Based Information—Provided by New Jersey Medical Libraries *(continued)*

	Yes	No	Unknown	Not Applicable
h. Preventative measures	( )	( )	( )	( )
i. Inpatient monitoring	( )	( )	( )	( )
j. Other (please specify)	( )	( )	( )	( )

Comments: _____

_____

_____

_____

_____

_____

9. Did the information you received contribute to your ability to AVOID any of the following for the PATIENT? (Check one answer for each item on the list.)

	Yes	No	Unknown	Not Applicable
a. Delay in diagnosis	( )	( )	( )	( )
b. Delay in treatment	( )	( )	( )	( )
c. Hospital admission	( )	( )	( )	( )
d. Patient mortality	( )	( )	( )	( )
e. Hospital acquired infection	( )	( )	( )	( )
f. Surgery	( )	( )	( )	( )
g. Injury to patient	( )	( )	( )	( )
h. Errors in dose or method of drug treatment	( )	( )	( )	( )
i. Inappropriate tests or procedures	( )	( )	( )	( )
j. Additional tests or procedures				
k. Additional outpatient visits	( )	( )	( )	( )

10. Has the information you received provided any of the following for YOURSELF? (Check one response for each item.)

	Yes	No
a. Reduced my professional time for research	( )	( )
b. Enhanced my explanations to patients about tests, etc.	( )	( )
c. Reduced my consultations with colleagues	( )	( )
d. Saved me money	( )	( )
e. Prevented liability	( )	( )
f. Other_____	( )	( )

Continued on next page

FIGURE 5 User Survey for Knowledge-Based Information— Provided by New Jersey Medical Libraries *(continued)*

Library Service Questions

11. Please express your satisfaction with the overall library services. Answer each question by circling the number on the scale most clearly describing your level of satisfaction.
    a. Speed of service 1   2   3   4   5   6
    b. Overall knowledge and
       ability of all staff 1   2   3   4   5   6
    c. Quality of resources available 1   2   3   4   5   6

12. If a fee is charged, what do you think is the average value for each service performed by the librarian at your request? (Please enter a dollar amount from $0 up.)
    a. One interlibrary loan . . . . ($)
    b. One computer search on Medline database . . . . ($)
    c. One article photocopy . . . . ($)

13. The following are examples of a physician's case experience using library information. Please describe a case where the LIBRARIAN played an important role in assisting you to deliver quality patient care.

Examples

Case 1. Life-Saving Benefits

Why search? "(I sought) case reports of a rare and usually fatal fungal infection and its suggested treatment."

How was the search helpful? "Based on information in these reports, I chose IV miconazole for a patient with a brain abscess due to this fungal infection."

What was the ultimate impact? "Patient has survived for two years and almost certainly would have died if this treatment had not been located."

Case 2. Application: Clinical Practice

Why Search? "I've done psychotherapy with several high-functioning autistic children who had a layer of depression that was significant to the extent of becoming suicidal. A psychiatrist told me about Aspeger's Syndrome that seemed to describe these children."

How was that information helpful? "The review board at our hospital tended to declare that autistic children are not cognitively able to be depressed. By showing them articles (found in the search) I have been able to convince them that depression does exist."

FIGURE 5 User Survey for Knowledge-Based Information—Provided by New Jersey Medical Libraries *(continued)*

What was the ultimate impact? "I was able to get more psychotherapeutic treatment for autistic, depressed children. Now I can put autism and depression on a child's DSM form and know the child will get more care."

Source: *Gratefully Yours,* March/April 1991

Your Case Example

_____
_____
_____
_____

Sources for survey:

A joint project of the New Jersey Hospital Association and the Health Sciences Library Association of New Jersey

Michele Volesko, Director of Library and Information Services
   New Jersey Hospital Association, Princeton, NJ

Claudia Allocco, Director of Library Services
   Valley Hospital, Ridgewood, NJ

James Delo, Chief Learning Resource Services
   Veterans Administration Medical Center, Lyons, NJ

Jane McCarthy, Retired, formerly Library Director
   Muhlenberg Regional Medical Center, Plainfield, NJ

Patricia May, Director of Library Services
   St. Joseph's Hospital and Medical Center, Paterson, NJ

Comparative Data/Information (IM.10–IM.10.3)

RELATED STANDARDS

In "Management of Information" Chapter:

IM.10 *The information-management function provides for the definition, capture, analysis, transmission, and reporting and/or use of comparative performance data and information, the comparability of which is based on national and state guidelines for data set parity and connectivity.*

IM.10.1 (Capped at Score 2)

A 1 2 3 4 5 NA   The organization uses external reference databases for comparative purposes.

IM.10.2 (Capped at Score 2)

A 1 2 3 4 5 NA   The organization contributes to external reference databases when required by law or regulation and/or when appropriate to the organization.

IM.10.3 (Capped at Score 2)

A 1 2 3 4 5 NA   The information-management function maintains the security and confidentiality of data and information when contributing to or using external databases.

In "Improving Organizational Performance" Chapter:

PI.2.1.4 (Capped at Score 2)

A 1 2 3 4 5 NA   [New processes are designed well. The design is based on] the performance of the processes and their outcomes in other organizations (such as information from reference databases).

PI.4.1.2.3 (Capped at Score 2)

A 1 2 3 4 5 NA   [The assessment process includes comparing data about] the organization's performance of processes and their outcomes to that of other organizations, including using reference databases.

The standards under IM.10 are closely linked with standards in the "Improving Organizational Performance" chapter. These standards require your organization to use external data and information in designing and assessing processes. Leaders and staff often use comparative information from reference databases in identifying deviations from expected patterns or trends and in setting priorities for improvement. When designing or improving a process, staff might also use benchmarking to identify "best practices."

IM.10 is also closely tied to the other standards in the "Management of Information" chapter. For example, IM.10.3 expands the requirements for confidentiality and security (IM.2) to data shared externally. It would be impossible to share data among organizations or with an external database without effective data linkages (IM.6). Finally, organizations must ensure uniformity in data capture and transmission (IM.3 and IM.5).

■ How Are These Standards Surveyed?

During the document review, surveyors will want to see a list of any external databases used by your organization for performance improvement. In addition, the surveyors will ask leaders and key staff members how they use comparative data and information gathered from a reference database(s).

All these standards are capped at a score of 2. Thus, your organization has a few years to comply with these requirements before it affects your accreditation decision.

COMMON QUESTIONS

Q. Must an organization formally consider the IMSystem?
A. The Joint Commission does not require organizations to consider the IMSystem. Participation in an outcomes measurement system such as the IMSystem is expected to be required when system data are used in evaluation activities associated with accreditation. This is not likely to occur before 1997. We expect your organization to consider any indicators that have been approved for use in the IMSystem as you make decisions on what to measure. (Appendix B should answer many of your questions regarding the IMSystem.)

Q. What comparative databases does the Joint Commission accept as meeting the intent of the standard?
A. The Joint Commission recognizes most sources of comparative data and information. Sources include state hospital associations (for example, financial, staffing efficiency studies); professional organizations; the Maryland Hospital Association Quality Indicator Project; and the Joint Commission's IMSystem. Within a large multihospital system that encompasses many similar hospitals (such as Department of Defense, Department of Veterans Affairs), a database containing data from hospitals within the system will permit each hospital to compare itself to other system hospitals. A comparative database should be relevant to an organization's scope of care, be risk adjusted, and provide feedback reports or information.

Performance Improvement (PI.3.4–PI.3.4.1.3)

RELATED STANDARDS

PI.3.4 (Capped at Score 2)

A 1 2 3 4 5 NA The organization measures the performance of processes in all the patient care and organizational functions identified in the *AMH*.

PI.3.4.1 *Processes measured on a continuing basis include those that*

PI.3.4.1.1 (No cap)

C 1 2 3 4 5 NA affect a large percentage of patients; and/or

PI.3.4.1.2 (No cap)

C 1 2 3 4 5 NA place patients at serious risk if not performed well, or performed when not indicated, or not performed when indicated; and/or

PI.3.4.1.3 (No cap)

C 1 2 3 4 5 NA   have been or are likely to be problem prone.

The improving organizational performance standards require that hospitals measure the performance of each function and chapter identified in the *AMH*. This includes the management of information function. Given the scope of this function, it is impossible to set up indicators to continually assess the entire function. Therefore, organizations need to identify key processes within the function that they will measure.

The standards identify three criteria that leaders and staff should use in determining which processes to measure on a ongoing basis:
- Whether the process affects a large percentage of the population;
- Whether the process places patients at serious risk if not performed well; and
- Whether the process is likely to be problem prone.

Other criteria might also be considered, such as costs, relation to strategic plans, and patient or user satisfaction. Application Example 3, on page 118, provides some tips on identifying ongoing measures.

An organization may also choose to design or redesign a particular process related to the management of information as a result of its needs assessment (IM.1). As part of these activities, your organization should set up measures to assess the success of this design or redesign effort.

■ How Are These Standards Surveyed?

The surveyors will review documentation to determine what processes related to the management of information are being measured. Later, in interviews with those staff members in charge of coordinating performance-improvement activities, surveyors will ask what methods were used to select these processes and how these processes are being monitored on a continual basis.

PI.3.4 is capped at a score of 2. Thus, organizations have some time to determine which processes regarding the management of information to continually assess. Organizations might already be measuring certain processes (for example, related to patient-specific information). As part of its needs assessment (IM.1.1), your organization should consider whether these measures are sufficient. To identify new measures, organizations should use the three criteria under standards PI.3.4.1.1 through PI.3.4.1.3.

COMMON QUESTIONS

Q. How many indicators are organizations expected to measure for the management of information function?
A. There are no longer numerical requirements on how many indicators organizations need to assess. To meet the requirement under PI.3.4, an organization should have at least one indicator that measures the performance of a process related to the management of information. However, your organization should measure as many indicators as is necessary to sufficiently evaluate the performance of the management of information function.

Q. Are organizations required to use the Joint Commission's cycle for improving performance in designing, measuring, assessing, and improving the management of information function?
A. No. Organizations are not required to use the cycle for improving performance outlined in Chapter 1. However, they are required to show evidence of compliance with the improving organizational performance standards. The cycle is intended to provide organizations with a roadmap for continually improving important functions in the *AMH*, and organizations should find it useful in guiding their improvement efforts.

FIGURE 6 Using the Cycle for Improving Performance

Design
After assessing its information needs, a health care network developed processes to link its clinical information systems. A representative team then developed a macroflow of the major processes to be designed. They also researched expert literature and comparative databases. Finally, using appropriate technologies, the team designed and implemented data linkages.

Measure
The team set up indicators to measure various aspects of the new processes. For example, one indicator measured timely access to data and information that are transmitted among entities. Data were collected for six months and fed into an internal database.

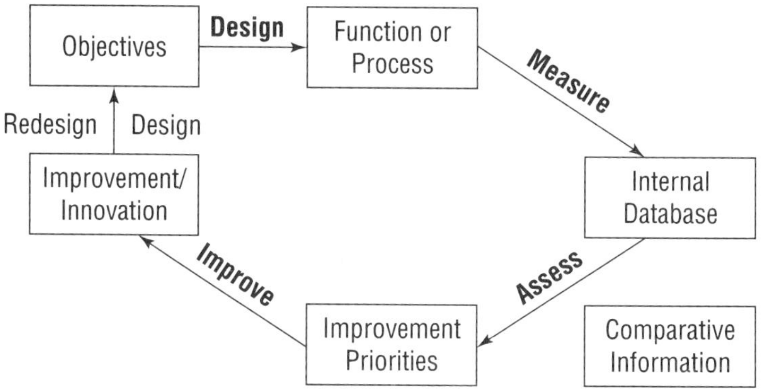

```
        Objectives  ──Design──►  Function or
           ▲                       Process
    Redesign │ Design                 │
           │                        Measure
    Improvement/                      ▼
    Innovation                   Internal
           ▲                     Database
         Improve                    │
           │                      Assess
       Improvement   ◄──        Comparative
        Priorities              Information
```

Improve
A subteam was assigned to investigate the problem. They found that it was a technical difficulty and were able to fix it. They then instituted corrective steps. The team continued to monitor the new process.

Assess
After six months, the team assessed the success of the new processes. Based on these findings, the team found that data transmission between home health and the hospital was much slower than between the clinics and the hospital.

The above example illustrates how the cycle for improving performance can guide a design effort. The example is brief and only intended to illustrate the cycle.

Figure 6, above, provides an example of how this cycle might apply when redesigning a particular management of information process.

Q. What are some examples of indicators used to measure the management of information function?
A. The following are some examples of process and outcome measures related to the management of information:

- Turnaround times of laboratory, radiology, or other reports;
- Accuracy of laboratory, radiology, or other reports;
- Billing turnaround (from discharge);
- Various accounts payable measures, such as number of days due or bill amount;
- Transcription turnaround trends;
- Number of "loose sheets" (reports that did not make it into the patient medical record during hospitalization);
- Turnaround time of "STAT" orders;
- Number of billing corrections;
- Rate of incorrect demographic information, such as patient age, in ambulatory records;
- Percentage of financial and other management reports that go unused;
- Frequency of manual operations or changes on computer-generated reports;
- Efficiency with which patient demographic data are aggregated;
- Timeliness by which financial information is available for operational decision making; and
- Timeliness of data transmission between infection control and safety functions.

This list is intended only to provide you with some measures that may be used to monitor the management of information function. Application Example 3, below, provides some tips on determining the indicators that are applicable to your organization.

APPLICATION EXAMPLE 3.

Identifying Measures for the Management of Information

One technique for selecting ongoing indicators is to use the Quality Cube (see Figure 7, page 119). On one axis of the cube are

FIGURE 7 The Quality Cube

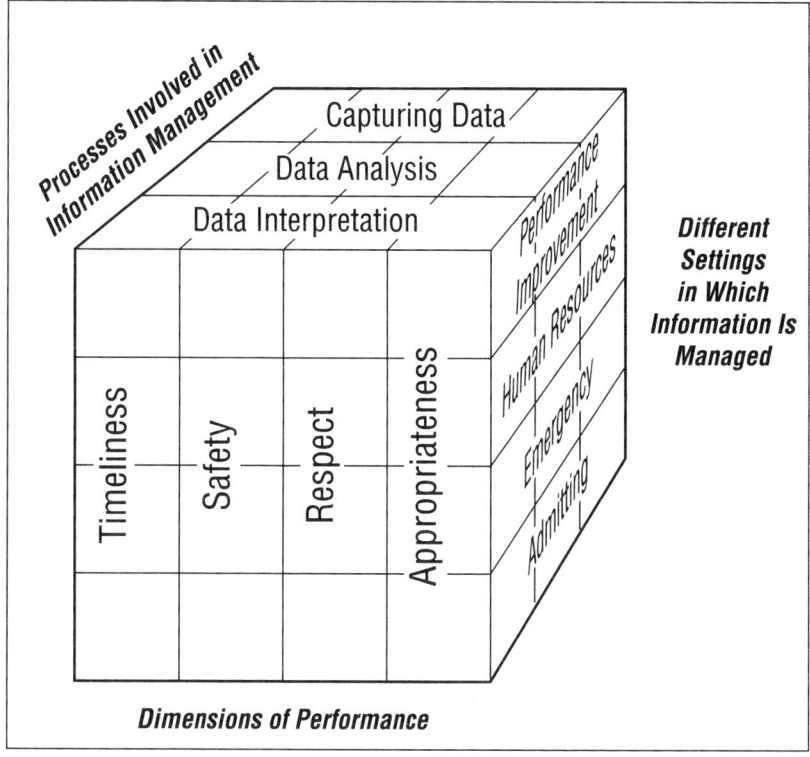

Organizations can use a three-dimensional axis in selecting indicators of performance.

dimensions of performance that were introduced on page 36 (for example, timeliness, appropriateness). Another axis lists the different processes involved in the management of information (for example, capturing data). The third axis lists the different settings in which information is managed (for example, admitting).

Using this three-dimensional matrix, you can identify "risk points" for the management of different types of information. For example, to measure the management of patient-based information, you might begin by asking "What are the most important dimensions of performance when managing patient-based data?" Timeliness might be one dimension chosen. Then, you might ask "Where in the organization is the timeliness of patient-based information important?" One area might be in the

FIGURE 8 Selection Grid for Choosing Performance Measures

Decision Factor / Area for Measurements							
High Volume							
High Risk							
Problem Prone							
Important to Organization's Mission							
Important to Patients							
Effect on Costs							
Total							

KEY TO SCORING: X = strong effect   x = 3
0 = some effect   0 = 2
- = weak effect   - = 1
  = no effect   = 0

This figure shows a selection grid that an organization could use to narrow areas for measurement. Staff members assign scores indicating how heavily the decision factor applies to each opportunity. Once the scores are totaled, staff members should indicate the priority of each possible measure within the listed factors.

operative suites. For example, you might identify the need to document the operative report in the medical record as an important aspect of performance because staff members who need to take care of a patient postoperatively must know what transpired during the operation.

From this activity, your organization might develop a long list of possible areas for measurement. Then you might use a selection matrix (Figure 8, page 120) to narrow the number to those areas that meet specific criteria and prioritize your measurement activities (for example, high volume, high risk, and problem prone).

CHAPTER 3

An Overview of the Survey Process

When the Joint Commission revised its standards to focus to a greater extent on the outcomes of important functions rather than the structures and processes organizations have in place (for example, policies and procedures), it also fundamentally changed the nature of its on-site surveys. The new survey process has been designed to assess the following issues:
- Are the correct processes performed?
- Are these processes performed well?
- Is the organization improving its performance?

To properly answer these questions, surveyors focus on assessing the *performance* of important functions across the organization. Rather than evaluating specific departments and services, the surveyors now concentrate on how well the various disciplines and hospital staff members work together to perform functions important to the patient, as well as the outcomes of those functions.

The new survey process for hospitals was implemented in January 1994, and will continue to be revised in 1995 and 1996. It was designed to support the patient-centered, performance-focused, functional orientation that was set forth in the revised accreditation manual. Other changes were also made to address complaints from the field concerning inconsistency across surveys and overemphasis on documentation, along with other issues. As a result, the surveys have become more interactive. Though some documentation review is still necessary, surveyors spend the majority of their time moving around your organization, talking with physicians and other staff members, and visiting patient care settings. The following pages describe the key changes that have been made to the hospital survey process.

■ Tailored to Your Organization

Prior to the survey, an organization liaison will work with your hospital to set a survey agenda and identify the most appropriate staff members to participate in the survey. Thus, the survey process will be tailored to reflect your organization's unique mission, scope of services, and processes. Since the agenda will be determined several weeks before the survey, it will be possible to schedule activities at times when medical and organization staff members are able to be present. Variations from the planned survey agenda will be infrequent and will only occur after the surveyors discuss the need for the schedule changes with organization leaders. For example, surveyors might need to follow up on certain issues later in the survey process.

■ More Consistency Across Surveys

Protocols have been developed to guide the survey process and increase consistency across surveys. These protocols identify data sources, describe methodologies, and provide probes, which surveyors use to review each important function in the *AMH*. To further promote consistency in the survey process, each survey team has an identified team leader. This leader is responsible for fostering consistent interpretation of the standards within a given team and from survey to survey.

■ Team-Based Approach to Surveying

In the past, the physician surveyor concentrated on medical staff-related reviews; the nurse surveyor dealt with nursing and other patient care issues; and the administrator surveyors handled reviews of governance, management, the physical plant, safety, and many ancillary department reviews. Once a surveyor had visited a specific department or completed a particular kind of review, it was often possible to score most or all of the applicable standards. Beginning in 1994, nothing is given a final score until the afternoon of the last day of the survey. For the most part, every surveyor is assessing all of the standards at all times. On the completion of the survey, the surveyors review all of their findings for each of the functional chapters in the *AMH* and decide as a team what the score should be for each standard, and the nature of the recommendation to be returned to the organization.

■ Interactive Process

Surveyors now spend considerably less time reviewing written materials and more time talking to staff members and patients, interviewing individuals and groups, and observing the delivery of care as they tour your organization. In addition to promoting surveyor-staff communication, the new survey process encourages staff from different disciplines and departments to interact with each other during the survey. Again, the standards recognize that most work in health care organizations is accomplished by teams of interdependent staff members whose individual efforts must be coordinated. Thus, many group interviews and discussions will be held throughout the survey. For example, physicians, nurses, and other health professionals will participate together in the visits to patient care settings.

Each surveyor also visits patient care units to observe the provision of care. The surveyors will meet with physicians and other care providers in those settings, whether they are inpatient units or treatment areas such as the emergency room, imaging, ambulatory clinics, rehabilitative services, and so forth. This component of the survey is designed to determine how well functions are actually carried out. It should also help surveyors gain a realistic perspective of the organization's day-to-day activities.

■ Longer Surveys

There is now greater interaction between surveyors and staff members and an increased integration of survey procedures to reflect the function-focused standards. This means that the new survey process will likely require more time than the previous process. Typically (except for hospitals with fewer than 50 beds), organizations that had a two-day survey in the past will now have a three-day survey.

■ Emphasis on Education

Surveyors have been encouraged to provide organizations with education and consultation concerning performance issues pertinent to the standards. Given their years of experience and the number of organizations they have surveyed, surveyors are able to share best practices from other organizations and advice on complying with standards.

■ Step-by-Step Through the Survey

Pre-Survey Activities

The survey process begins when an organization applies for an accreditation survey or is due for its triennial survey. Six weeks before the survey, your organization will be assigned a Joint Commission liaison responsible for coordinating your survey and setting its agenda.

As part of presurvey planning, each organization will be asked to identify those staff members involved in the management of information. The organization will also be asked to identify data sources regarding the management of information. To facilitate the surveyors' review, staff members are asked to create an index that cross-references each document to the specific standard it addresses (for example, assessment of information needs). Staff members are also asked to organize their documents in clearly marked binders and to place tabs throughout the binders indicating the standards number(s) to which the materials pertain.

The survey team, composed of at least a physician, an administrator, a nurse, and often other specialist surveyors, receives a "presurvey management report" packet to help orient team members to your organization. The packet includes the customized survey agenda, a copy of the previous accreditation survey report, information regarding any complaints about your organization received by the Joint Commission, and survey documents. One surveyor is designated "team leader" to facilitate on-site survey activities and act as a first-line contact for your organization.

All surveyors assess your organization's compliance with the management of information standards. They will review documents, interview key staff members, review medical records, and observe how information is managed as they tour the organization. Certain aspects will be surveyed by particular surveyors (for example, the administrator surveyor will conduct the management of information group interview).

The following paragraphs walk you through a typical survey. The discussion does not necessarily represent the order of your survey's progression because, as discussed above, your organization's survey agenda will be determined with your organization liaison (see Figure 9, page 128, for a sample agenda). The discussion focuses primarily on those activities in which the management of information function is reviewed. Table 8, page 132, also provides "probes" that surveyors use to review the management of information function. Your organization might find this list useful in preparing for the survey.

FIGURE 9 Survey Agenda: Four-Day Survey—1995 Hospital Accreditation Services Survey

DAY 1	
All Surveyors	
8:30–8:45 AM	Opening Conference
8:45–9:15 AM	Overview of Organization's Performance-Improvement Approach
9:15–11:45 AM	Document Review Session
11:45–12:30 PM	Leadership Interview
12:30–1:00 PM	Lunch

Physician Surveyor	Nurse Surveyor	Administrator Surveyor
1:15–2:15 PM Patient Care Setting Visit[1]	1:15–2:15 PM Patient Care Setting Visit[1]	1:15–2:15 PM Patient Care Setting Visit[1]
2:15–3:15 PM Patient Care Setting Visit[1]	2:15–3:15 PM Operating Room Visit	2:15–2:45 PM Patient and Family Education Interview
3:15–4:00 PM Patient Care Setting Visit[1]	3:15–4:00 PM Patient Care Setting Visit[1]	2:45–3:15 PM Ethics Interview
		3:15–4:00 PM Patient Care Setting Visit[1]

All Surveyors
4:00–4:30 PM Survey Team Meeting

This is a sample of a four-day accreditation survey. Your organization's agenda will be determined with your organizational liaison.

FIGURE 9 Survey Agenda: Four-Day Survey—1995 Hospital Accreditation Services Survey *(continued)*

DAY 2

All Surveyors

8:30–8:45 AM Daily Briefing

Physician Surveyor	Nurse Surveyor	Administrator Surveyor
8:45–10:00 AM Imaging Services Visit[2] 10:00–11:00 AM Patient Care Setting Visit[1] 11:00–12:00 AM Patient Care Setting Visit[1]	8:45–10:00 AM Patient Care Setting Visit[1] 10:00–11:00 AM Patient Care Setting Visit[1] 11:00–12:00 AM Continuum of Care Interview	8:45–12:00 AM Building Tour[3]

All Surveyors

12:00–12:30 PM Lunch
12:45–1:45 PM Medication/Nutrition Care Interview

Physician Surveyor	Nurse Surveyor	Administrator Surveyor
1:45–3:00 PM Emergency Services Visit	1:45–3:00 PM Patient Care Setting Visit[1]	1:45–2:15 PM Pharmacy Services Visit 2:15–2:30 PM Admitting Services Visit 2:30–3:00 PM Resource Center Visit 3:00–4:00 PM Rehabilitation Services Visit

Physician and Nurse Surveyors

3:00–4:00 PM Operative and Other Invasive Procedures Interview

All Surveyors

4:00–4:30 PM Survey Team Meeting

Continued on next page

FIGURE 9 Survey Agenda: Four-Day Survey—1995 Hospital Accreditation Services Survey *(continued)*

DAY 3

All Surveyors

8:30–8:45 AM Daily Briefing

Physician Surveyor	Nurse Surveyor	Administrator Surveyor
8:45–9:45 AM Pathology and Clinical Laboratory Services Visit[4]	8:45–10:00 AM Patient Care Setting Visit[1]	8:45–9:45 AM Chief Executive Officer/ Strategic Planning and Resource Allocation Interview
9:45–11:15 AM Medical Staff Credentials Review	10:00–11:00 AM Nursing Leadership Interview	9:45–11:45 AM Review of Environment of Care Documents
11:15–12:30 PM Medical Staff Leadership Interview	11:00–12:00 AM Patient Care Setting Visit[1]	11:45–12:15 PM Lunch
12:30–1:30 PM Lunch: Medical Staff Conference (optional)	12:00–12:30 PM Lunch	12:30–1:15 PM Information Management Interview
1:45–3:00 PM Patient Care Setting Visit[1]	12:45–1:45 PM Infection Control Interview	1:15–2:00 PM Patient Care Setting Visit[1]
	1:45–3:00 PM Patient Care Setting Visit[1]	2:00–3:00 PM Hospital Department Directors Interview
		3:00–4:00 PM Human Resources Function Interview

Physician and Nurse Surveyors

3:00–4:00 PM Medical Record Review

All Surveyors

4:00–4:30 PM Survey Team Meeting

FIGURE 9 Survey Agenda: Four-Day Survey—1995 Hospital Accreditation Services Survey *(continued)*

DAY 4

All Surveyors

9:00–10:00 AM 8:30–9:00 AM Daily Briefing
              Competence Assessment Process Review

Physician Surveyor	Nurse Surveyor	Administrator Surveyor
10:00–11:00 AM Performance-Improvement Group Interview	10:00–11:00 AM Performance-Improvement Group Interview	10:00–11:00 AM Performance-Improvement Group Interview

All Surveyors

11:00–12:00 AM Performance-Improvement Coordinating Group Interview
12:00–12:30 PM Lunch
12:30–3:00 PM   Team Meeting to Integrate Survey Findings
3:15–4:15 PM   Chief Executive Officer Exit Conference

[1]Includes inpatient units and other sites where care is rendered, including ambulatory settings and anesthetizing locations, other than those specifically named in the survey agenda.
[2]Includes diagnostic radiology, nuclear medicine, and radiation oncology, as appropriate.
[3]Includes visits to kitchen, storage, central supply, and laundry, if applicable.
[4]Includes survey of the use of blood and blood components (PI.3.4.2.3).

TABLE 8 Survey Probes for the Management of Information Function

Note: The following issues may be addressed at the survey activities listed below. Although stated in question form, these "probes" are not "canned questions" and will be tailored to each organization based on surveyors' review of organizational documents and previous survey activities.

Leadership Interview
- Has there been an assessment of the information-management needs of the organization? How are information systems planned to meet the information needs of the organization? (IM.1 through IM.1.1.2)
- What types of aggregate data are available to leaders of the organization in support of managerial decisions, operations, and performance measurement, assessment, and improvement activities relating to patient care activities? (IM.8)

Medical Staff Leadership Interview
- Is the format and organization of the medical record well designed for user's needs? (IM.5 through IM.5.1)
- Are medical records accessible at all necessary times (for example, unplanned ambulatory and emergency service needs)? (IM.5 through IM.5.1)
- Are the results of diagnostic tests available to practitioners in a timely fashion? (IM.5 through IM.5.1)
- What is the system for the management of practitioner-specific information for licensed independent practitioners? Is it adequate to meet the needs for this type of information in the reappointment and review or revision of clinical privileges? (IM.8.1.10)
- What types of aggregate data are available to the leaders of the organization in support of managerial decisions, operations, improvement activities, and patient care functions? (IM.8)
- What access is available to knowledge-based information that may be required in patient care activities, research, and other clinical activities? (IM.9 through IM.9.4.1)
- What use is made of the comparative database or information gathered from the reference database(s) in which the organization participates? (IM.10 through IM.10.3)

Nursing Leadership Interview
- Is the format and organization of the medical record well designed for user's needs? (IM.5 through IM.5.1)
- Are patient records accessible at all necessary times (for example, unplanned ambulatory and emergency services needs)? (IM.5 through IM.5.1)
- Are the results of diagnostic tests available to practitioners in a timely fashion? (IM.5 through IM.5.1)

TABLE 8 Survey Probes for the Management of Information Function *(continued)*

- What is the system for the management of practitioner-specific information for licensed independent practitioners? Is it adequate to meet the needs for this type of information? (IM.8.1.10)
- What types of aggregate data are available to the leaders of the organization in support of managerial decisions, operations, improvement activities, and patient care functions? (IM.8)
- What access is available to knowledge-based information that may be required in patient care activities, research, and other clinical activities? (IM.9 through IM.9.4.1)
- What use is made of a comparative database or information gathered from the reference database(s) in which the organization participates? (IM.10 through IM.10.3)

CEO/Strategic Planning and Resource Allocation Interview
- What types of aggregate data are available to the leaders of the organization in support of managerial decisions, operations, and performance measurement, assessment, and improvement activities, relating to patient care activities? (IM.8)
- What coding and retrieval systems are used for financial information? (IM.8.1.7)
- What resources are provided to meet the organization's needs for knowledge-based information or literature? (IM.9.1)

Performance Improvement Coordinating Group Interview
- What are the linkages among information management processes related to important patient care and organizational functions in the organization? (IM.6.2)
- What mechanisms are in place to develop data and information for performance improvement activities? (IM.8.1.8 through IM.8.1.9)

Information Management Interview (group interview)
- Describe the system for making information available to those who need it in carrying out their responsibilities. Who is responsible for ensuring the availability of needed information? (IM.1 through IM.1.1.2)
- Describe the planning process for managing patient-specific and aggregate clinical data. (IM.1 through IM.1.1.2)
- What measures are in place to ensure confidentiality, security, integrity of patient health and other vital records? (IM.2 through IM.2.3)
- What uniform data definitions and methods for capturing data are in place? (IM.3 through IM.3.3)
- Describe the means in place to permit integration of data across information systems in the organization. (IM.6 through IM.6.3)

Continued on next page

TABLE 8 Survey Probes for the Management of Information Function (continued)

- What types of aggregate data are available to the leaders of the organization in support of managerial decisions, operations, and performance measurement, assessment, and improvement activities relating to patient care activities? (IM.8)
- What use is made of the comparative data and information gathered from the reference database(s) in which the organization participates? (IM.10 through IM.10.3)

Interviews With Hospital Department Director and All Department Service Directors
- What education have you had in the principles of information management? (IM.4)
- What types of aggregate data are available to department directors in support of managerial decisions, operations, and performance measurement, assessment, and improvement activities relating to patient care activities? (IM.8)
- Describe how knowledge-based information resources are made available to all those who need them, are authoritative, and are up to date. (IM.9.4 through IM.9.4.1; IM.6.3)

Medical Record Review
- What are the organization's policies regarding the timely completion of medical records (for example, when is a record delinquent)? (IM.7.7.2) How many records are delinquent at the time of the survey? (Complete form.)
- Are medical records available as needed on a 24-hour basis? (IM.5 through IM.5.1) What is the process for their access?
- What are the organization's policies regarding:
  - Completion of the medical history and physical examination after admission?
  - Use of medical history and physical examination information gathered in physician offices within 30 days prior to admission?
  - Extent of history and assessment that is required when a patient is readmitted to the organization?
  - Timely reporting of autopsy findings? (IM.7.7 through IM.7.7.2)
- What issues have been identified as a result of the medical record review activity of the organization? How have opportunities to improve or problems been addressed? (IM.3.3.1)
- What use is made of the comparative data and information gathered from the reference database(s) in which the organization participates? (IM.10 through IM.10.3)
- Describe the means in place to permit integration of data across information systems in the organization. (IM.6 through IM.6.3)

TABLE 8 Survey Probes for the Management of Information Function (continued)

- What types of aggregate data are available to department directors in support of managerial decisions, operations, and performance measurement, assessment, and improvement activities relating to patient care activities? (IM.8)
- Describe the coding and retrieval system for medical records by diagnosis and procedure. (IM.8.1.5)

Pharmaceutical Services Visit
- What means are in place to identify the signatures of all practitioners authorized to prescribe medications? (IM.8.1.1.1)
- Is there a listing of all Drug Enforcement Administration numbers for those authorized to prescribe? (IM.6.1.1.2)
- What types of aggregate data are available to department directors in support of managerial decisions, operations, and performance measurement, assessment, and improvement activities, relating to patient care activities? (IM.8)
- Is access to poison-control information readily available to the pharmacy, medical, and nursing staff? (IM.9.5)
- Is the organization formulary and/or drug list readily available to the professional staff who use it? (IM.9.6)

Resource Center Visit
- Describe the process of assessing the knowledge-based information needs of the organization with special attention to
  - the need for accessibility and timeliness
  - the need to link with appropriate external database(s) and information networks; and
  - the need to link with the organization's internal information systems. (IM.9.2 through IM.9.2.1.3)
- Describe how knowledge-based information resources are made available to all those who need them, are authoritative, and are up-to-date. (IM.9.1 through IM.9.4.1; IM.6.3)
- What types of aggregate data are available to department directors in support of managerial decisions, operations, and performance measurement, assessment, and improvement activities relating to patient care activities? (IM.8.1.11)

Visits to Patient Care Settings
Patient care setting includes inpatient units and other areas where patients' needs are assessed and care is provided (for example, emergency room, rehabilitation).
- What types of aggregate data are available to staff in the unit in support of managerial decisions, operations, and assessment and improvement activities? (IM.8)

Continued on next page

TABLE 8 Survey Probes for the Management of Information Function *(continued)*

- Is there appropriate access to poison-control information and the organization formulary and/or drug list by those in need of the information? (IM.9.5 through IM.9.6)
- Describe how knowledge-based information resources are available to all those who need them, are authoritative, and are up to date. (IM.9.4 through IM.9.4.1; IM.6.3)

Open and Closed Record Review
- Presence or absence of entries and their adequacy in the medical record (IM.3.3.1 through IM.3.3.1.2; IM.7.2 through IM.7.9.3) (See medical record review forms and description of medical record interviews.)
- All relevant requested inpatient, ambulatory care, and emergency care records of the patient are assembled when the patient is receiving care. (IM.7.10 through IM.7.10.1)

Medical Staff Credentials Review
- The use of data and information regarding the performance of licensed independent practitioners, as defined in the "Medical Staff" chapter (IM.8.1.10)

Visits to Other Sites of Care (emergency, outpatient, and so forth)
- What is the process to maintain the control register? Are the appropriate items included in the content? (IM.8.1.6.1)

Introductory Sessions

Every survey begins with a brief *Opening Conference*. This is simply an opportunity for organization leaders and the survey team to become acquainted. During the conference, the survey agenda is clarified and adjusted, if necessary; however, nothing specific to the management of information function is discussed. The Opening Conference is followed by a 30-minute presentation of your organization's performance improvement activities, which is a new survey activity in 1995. This activity is intended to orient surveyors to your organization's approach to performance improvement.

Document Review

Following the opening conference, the survey team privately reviews the key documents that your organization was asked to have available. These include bylaws, various planning documents, policies, procedures, and rules and regulations. The initial document review helps the survey team become familiar with your organization's structure for providing patient care, and helps them begin to assess standards compliance and prepare for the interactive survey that follows. In addition, the surveyors will assess specific documents related to the management of information standards (see Table 9, page 138). They will also review your organization's last four calendar quarters of medical record reviews (see also "Medical Record Interview," page 146).

Leadership Interview

The surveyors meet jointly with senior leaders, including the chief executive officer, chairman of the governing body, medical staff leader, nurse executive, and performance improvement director on the first day of the survey. This interview is conducted primarily to determine the level of communication and collaboration among leaders and assess how well they comply with the leadership standards. Surveyors will ask if leaders have defined and communicated a common vision, mission, and strategic plan throughout the organization, and have provided an appropriate framework for reaching the goals set forth.

Because information plays such a vital role in carrying out an organization's strategic plans, the surveyors will ask leaders questions concerning the management of information function. For example, leaders might be asked to describe how they have collaborated to address the organization's information needs. Surveyors might also ask about what types of aggregate data are available to leaders to support managerial decisions, and operations, along with performance measurement, assessment, and improvement activities.

TABLE 9 Information Management Documents Typically Requested for Document Review Session

Note: The official list of documents requested for document review is included in the "Guidelines for Survey" mailed to your organization several weeks before survey.

- Documents, minutes, reports, and the like that evidence assessment of the needs of the organization and its components for access to internal and external information and plans to meet those needs (IM.1 through IM.1.1.2)
- Policies relating to the need for and appropriate levels of security and confidentiality of data and information (IM.2.1)
- Organization and medical staff policies relating to when patient records may be removed from the organization's jurisdiction (IM.2.2.1)
- Evidence of the presence of a mechanism to preserve confidentiality of patient-specific data and information identified as sensitive or requiring extraordinary means to preserve patient privacy (for example, psychiatric records) (IM.2.2.2)
- Evidence of the mechanism to safeguard records/information against loss, destruction, and tampering, and from access or use by unauthorized individuals (IM.2.3)
- Data policies, standards, and procedures relating to uniform data definitions and uniform methods for capturing data (IM.3 through IM.3.3)
- Policies and procedures relating to the content of the medical record, its completeness, accuracy, and timely completion (IM.3.3.1 through IM.3.3.1.2; IM.7.2 through IM.7.3.2)
- Reports or minutes of the group responsible for the performance of the quarterly review of medical records for quality of documentation and timely completion (for example, Medical Record Review Committee) for the most recent 12 months (IM.3.3.1 through IM.3.3.1.2)
- Staff education outlines, and so forth, regarding the management of information, and their relationship to the needs of individual members of the staff (IM.4)
- Policy regarding the length of time that medical records are retained (IM.6.1)
- Policies regarding the content of the medical record (IM.7.2 through IM.7.3.2)
- The policy or procedure regarding which procedures and treatments require informed consent documented in the medical record (IM.7.2.10)
- Policies and procedures regarding the recording of operative reports (IM.7.4.2 through IM.7.4.2.2)
- Policies that define the content and timeliness of a completed medical record (IM.7.7.2)

TABLE 9 Information Management Documents Typically Requested for Document Review Session *(continued)*

- Medical staff rules and regulations regarding verbal orders for medications. Who must authenticate such verbal orders? (IM.7.8 through IM.7.8.2.1)
- Policies and procedures regarding the use of rubber-stamp signatures or computer keys to authenticate entries in the patient health record (IM.7.9.2 through IM.7.9.2.1)
- Description of the system that is in place to assemble all required inpatient, ambulatory care, and emergency care records regarding the patient when care is received, including unscheduled ambulatory and emergency visits (IM.7.10 through IM.7.10.1)
- Documents that reflect the assessment of the organization's needs to use aggregate data and information (IM.8.1)
- Evidence of the organization's assessment of its needs for knowledge-based information (for example, written plan, surveys of needs, notes or minutes of meetings) (IM.9.2.1)
- A list of what external comparative databases are used by the organization in its performance improvement processes (IM.10 through IM.10.3)

Visits to Patient Care Settings

Visits to patient care settings,* including inpatient units, constitute a significant component of the survey process. These visits will concentrate on your organization's performance of important functions identified in the *AMH*, which includes the management of information. The units that surveyors visit will depend on your presurvey arrangements.

Members of the survey team will conduct these visits individually. Thus, the nurse surveyor might visit one unit, while the administrator visits another. There will be some variation in emphasis during visits to different units due to the mission and scope of care on that unit. However, on all units, surveyors will address to some degree all the patient-focused and organizational functions.

---

* "Patient care setting" refers to inpatient units, ambulatory clinics, emergency room, imaging, rehabilitation, anesthetizing locations, and any other sites where patients receive care.

Visit to Inpatient Units. As described below, each inpatient unit visit will follow the same general format.

Orientation to the Unit. The surveyor begins each visit by explaining the purpose of the visit to the unit manager(s) and any other staff. To become familiar with the unit, the surveyor will look at a list of patients and diagnoses. He or she may also have other background questions, such as admission criteria, common diagnoses on the unit, and so forth.

Tour of the Unit. Unit managers will be expected to give the surveyor a tour of the unit. During this time, the surveyor will primarily observe issues related to infection control, the environment of care (for example, hazardous materials, life safety), and patient rights issues. They also look at bulletin boards, posters, and so forth for evidence of communication, staff development, and performance-improvement activities.

Staff Conference. After touring the unit, the surveyor will sit down with the unit manager(s), physicians, nurses, social workers, and representatives of other disciplines that provide care on that unit and have been scheduled to participate. The surveyor will ask staff various questions related to different functions in the *AMH*. For example, with regard to the management of information, the surveyor might ask caregivers if they have access to the different types of information they need to carry out activities (for example, aggregate information for planning and decision-making purposes, clinical and scientific information required for delivering patient care).

Review of Open Medical Records. This review is typically done during the staff conference so that appropriate caregivers can participate in the review process. One or more patient records will be selected for review by the surveyor. Criteria for selection include:

- The diagnosis or procedure for which the patient was admitted to the unit clearly reflects the primary mission of the unit. (When the unit serves as an overflow unit for certain types of patients usually cared for on a specialty unit, one of the records may reflect the overflow function of the unit.)
- The care provided to the patient includes care provided by the disciplines that will be present in the staff conference.
- For a patient who is close to discharge or who has been hospitalized for a long period of time, there is sufficient documentation in the record for substantive discussion and/or evidence in the record of discharge planning and of patient and family teaching.

Essentially, the surveyor will walk through the medical record with staff members, addressing all functions that are pertinent to the unit being visited. Key issues assessed generally include the following:

- Assessment and reassessment of patients, such as involvement of all appropriate disciplines and hand-offs from one health care professional to another;
- Care of patients, as appropriate to the unit;
- Education of patients and family;
- Discharge planning;
- Management of information, especially issues addressed under standard IM.7; and
- Patient rights issues, do-not-resuscitate orders, or withdrawal of support.

In relation to the management of information, the surveyor will be interested in the content of the medical record and whether it reflects the care provided. The surveyor will also assess the completeness of the medical record. For example, are all relevant and requested inpatient, ambulatory care, and emergency care records of the patient assembled? (See also "Medical Record Interview," page 146.)

Brief Conversation with Patient and/or Family. After the staff conference and with the approval of the patient, the surveyor will have a brief conversation with one of the patients whose record is chosen for review and/or with his or her family members. The surveyor will talk with the patient and/or observe the care being provided. This conversation will provide the surveyor with an opportunity to assess how staff members relate to the patient and/or family as well as how privacy and confidentiality issues are handled.

Visits to Other Care Areas. In addition to visiting inpatient units, surveyors will visit the following areas of the hospital where patient needs are assessed and care is provided. These include:
- Anesthetizing areas, including the operating room, same-day surgery (if separate from main operating room), endoscopy, cardiac catheterization, labor and delivery and dental clinics;
- Rehabilitative services, including alcohol and drug dependency services, as well as physical therapy;
- Emergency services;
- Distinct ambulatory care clinics; and
- Imaging services, including diagnostic radiology, nuclear medicine, physical rehabilitation, and radiation oncology.

These visits generally follow the same format as the visits to patient care settings, except there may not be a conversation with a patient and/or their family members. The surveyor will talk to the department director and appropriate staff, tour the area, and review one or more open records, if available. With regard to the management of information, the surveyor will be interested in whether directors and staff have access to appropriate data and information. Specific questions will reflect the treatment area visited. For example, in the emergency room, the surveyor will ask about the process in place for maintaining the control register.

Management of Information Interview

At a prearranged time during the survey, the administrator surveyor will meet with key individuals involved in the management of information. This meeting lasts approximately 45 minutes. Participants should include:

- Chief information officer, if applicable;
- Information systems director, if applicable;
- The manager of the resource center or librarian;
- The director of medical records; and
- Other key individuals involved in the integration and use of information in the organization, if applicable.

Other staff members may also participate at the discretion of the organization.

During this meeting, the surveyor hopes to gain a better understanding of your organization's planning processes and approaches to the management of information. The surveyor has already read through relevant documents related to your management of information processes. However, he or she may need to clarify some information. The surveyor will also be concerned that the processes described in your documents match what is actually occurring. For example, is the needs assessment described in your information plan completed? What are the results? How are these results being used to set priorities?

During the meeting, the surveyor will ask the group to describe your information-planning activities, including the needs assessment. The surveyor will also focus on key issues covered under Standards IM.1 through IM.10, including the following:

- The system to make information available to users;
- How information needs are assessed and accommodated in the organization's planning process;
- How confidentiality, security, and integrity of information are assured;
- The mechanisms in place to develop and monitor the use of uniform data definitions and capture needed data;
- The means used to integrate information across information systems;
- The types of aggregate data and information available to those responsible for managing organizational activities; and
- The use the organization makes of comparative data and information.

Other Interviews

The surveyors conduct many other interviews with various leaders, department managers, and staff. These include the following:
- Chief Executive Officer and Strategic Planning and Resource Allocation;
- Ethics mechanisms;
- Human resources function (expanded in 1995);
- Infection control;
- Continuum of care (new in 1995);
- Medical records;
- Medical staff leadership;
- Nursing leadership;
- Performance-improvement teams; and
- Performance-improvement coordinating group.

The management of information will probably be brought up in some fashion in all these interviews. In general, surveyors will ask various leaders and staff whether they have appropriate access to the various types of data and information (patient-based, aggregate, knowledge-based, and comparative) they need to carry out patient care, make managerial decisions, carry out performance-improvement activities, and conduct research, if applicable. They will also ask about the education that leaders and staff have had in the principles of management of information. Figure 10, page 145, provides some specific issues that surveyors may focus on when interviewing these various groups or individuals.

Building Tour

During the building tour, the administrator surveyor visits non-patient care areas, such as admitting, food service, central sterile supply, and laundry. The main purpose of the tour is to assess issues related to life safety management. The surveyor may also visit some patient care settings to address structural or design issues above the ceiling tiles. The surveyor is accompanied by the organization's safety officer and/or engineer.

FIGURE 10 Information Management Standards to Be Discussed with Applicable Departments and/or Services

In preparation for interviews regarding the management of information standards, departments, or services should be prepared to respond to questions related to the standards indicated by an "X".

Please note: The surveyor may ask questions related to other standards not listed in the table as indicated by the survey

A = Leadership
B = Medical Staff
C = Nursing Leadership
D = Chief Executive Officer
E = Medical Records
F = P.T.S.M
G = Pharmacy Services
H = Resource Center
I = Quality Improvement Council
J = Information Managment
K = Emergency Services
L = Ambulatory Care
M = All Directors

IM STANDARD	A	B	C	D	E	F	G	H	I	J	K	L	M
1.–1.1.2	X												
2.–2.3										X			
3.–3.3										X			
5.–5.1		X	X							X			
6.1.1.2							X						
6.2					X				X				
6.3								X		X			X
6.–6.3					X					X			
7.2					X								
7.7–7.7.2					X								
8	X	X	X	X	X	X	X	X		X			X
8.1.1.1							X						
8.1.5							X						
8.1.6.1							X				X		
8.1.10												X	
8.1.8–8.1.9									X				
8.1.2–8.1.2.3						X							

This grid pinpoints specific standards surveyors will discuss during interviews with departments and/or services.

Medical Record Interview

Prior to the survey, your organization will be sent materials related to the medical record interview, including a medical record form (see Figure 11, page 147) and the tally for closed medical record forms (see Figure 12, page 151). At the end of the document review session, the survey team leader will present a list of requested closed medical records. This list will be based on the protocol for the medical records interview (see Figure 13, page 158). The survey team may also specify additional selection criteria (for example, specification of time frames).

While the surveyors carry out other survey activities, staff members from your organization will need to retrieve the requested closed medical records and do the following:

- Prepare a list of the medical record numbers on the organization's letterhead;
- Complete one closed medical record form for each record; and
- Complete the tally of closed medical record forms.

Staff must then present this information at the scheduled medical record review interview. This interview is conducted by the physician and nurse surveyors and includes the following staff:

- Administration and/or management;
- Health information management;
- Medical staff;
- Nursing;
- Staff members who complete the closed medical record forms and tally, and others in the organization who are responsible for the quality of medical record documentation; and
- Representatives from the organizational oversight group(s), such as a medical record committee or whatever mechanism is used to review the content of medical records on a regular basis.

FIGURE 11 Closed Medical Record Form

> ### *Introduction*
> Medical records are important data sources in the accreditation survey. During the survey, hospitals are required to review closed medical records, using the attached Closed Medical Record Form and based on the survey team record request.
>
> The closed medical records and their corresponding Closed Medical Record Forms must be completed and presented to the surveyor at the Medical Record Interview.
>
> Please follow the directions provided to complete the Closed Medical Record Form. Please direct any questions about the form to the surveyors.
>
> ### *Please Note:*
> ***The attached closed medical record form is required to be used.***
>
> | Item # | Standard # | | Y | N | NA |
> |---|---|---|---|---|---|
> | | | **History and Physical** | | | |
> | ____ | PE.1.7.1 | H and P completed within 24 hours of admission | ___ | ___ | ___ |
> | ____ | IM.7.2.6 | Diagnosis/impression recorded on H and P | ___ | ___ | ___ |
> | ____ | IM.7.2.7 | Reason admitted is documented | ___ | ___ | ___ |
> | ____ | IM.7.2.8 | Treatment plans documented in H and P | ___ | ___ | ___ |
> | | | **Orders** | | | |
> | ____ | IM.7.9 | All orders are dated and authenticated | ___ | ___ | ___ |
> | ____ | IM.7.8.1 | Verbal orders authenticated within organization's required time frame | ___ | ___ | ___ |
> | ____ | IM.7.9 | Housestaff orders are countersigned | ___ | ___ | ___ |
> | | | **Education** | | | |
> | | | (patient and family, as applicable) | | | |
> | ____ | PF.2.1 | Assessment of needs, abilities, and readiness | ___ | ___ | ___ |
> | ____ | PF.2.1.1 | Assessment of culture, religion, and limitations | ___ | ___ | ___ |
> | ____ | PF.2.2.1 | Education about safe and effective use of meds | ___ | ___ | ___ |
> | ____ | PF.2.2.2 | Education about safe and effective use of equipment | ___ | ___ | ___ |
> | ____ | PF.2.2.3 | Education for diet, nutrition, drug or food interaction | ___ | ___ | ___ |
> | ____ | PF.2.2.4 | Instructed about rehab techniques | ___ | ___ | ___ |
> | ____ | PF.2.2.5 | Instructed about community resources | ___ | ___ | ___ |
> | ____ | PF.4.2 | Educational process was interdisciplinary | ___ | ___ | ___ |
>
> Continued on next page

The medical records staff will complete and present this form to surveyors at the medical record interview.

FIGURE 11 Closed Medical Record Form *(continued)*

Item #	Standard #		Y	N	NA
_____	PF.2.2.6	Educated about when and how to obtain further care	___	___	___
_____	PF.3	Educated on discharge instructions	___	___	___
		Assessment of Patients			
_____	TX.3.4.1	Monitoring of meds' effect on the patient includes assessment based on collective observations including the patient's own perception	___	___	___
_____	PE.1.1	Need for care and/or treatment, type of care and further assessment is determined and documented	___	___	___
_____	PE.1.1	Physical, social, and psychological assessments are documented	___	___	___
		Scope and/or intensity of further assessment is determined by:	___	___	___
_____	PE.1.2.1	patient diagnosis;	___	___	___
_____	PE.1.2.2	treatment setting;	___	___	___
_____	PE.1.2.3	patient desire for treatment; and	___	___	___
_____	PE.1.2.4	patient response to previous treatment	___	___	___
_____	PE.1.3	Need for nutritional assessment is determined	___	___	___
_____	PE.1.4	Need for functional assessment is determined	___	___	___
_____	PE.1.6	Need for discharge planning is assessed	___	___	___
_____	TX.4.1	TPN requirement is based on assessment	___	___	___
_____	TX.4.2	Orders for TPN are based on assessment	___	___	___
		History and Physical			
_____	IM.7.2.15	Is present in the medical record	___	___	___
_____	PE.2.1	Is completed at specified times in the course of treatment	___	___	___
_____	PE.2.2	Is done to determine the patient's response to treatment	___	___	___
_____	PE.2.3	Is done when there is a significant change in patient's condition	___	___	___
_____	PE.2.4	Is done when there is a significant change in patient's diagnosis	___	___	___
_____	PE.3	Assessment data are integrated to identify and prioritize patient's needs for care and/or treatment	___	___	___
_____	PE.3.1	Care and/or treatment decisions are based on patient needs and/or priorities	___	___	___
		Operative and Invasive Procedures			
_____	PE.1.8	Preop. H and P and diagnosis is recorded	___	___	___
_____	IM.7.4.1	- by licensed independent practitioner	___	___	___
_____	PE.1.8.1	Preanesthesia assessment (for example, risk, ASA) is documented	___	___	___

FIGURE 11 Closed Medical Record Form *(continued)*

Item #	Standard #		Y	N	NA
_____	TX.2.1	Preop plan for anesthesia is recorded	___	___	___
_____	PE.1.8.2	Patient determined to be appropriate anesthesia candidate	___	___	___
_____	PE.1.8.2.1	- by licensed independent practitioner	___	___	___
_____	TX.5.3.1	Nursing care plan recorded preop.	___	___	___
_____	TX.5.3.2	A procedure and/or op plan is recorded preop.	___	___	___
_____	PE.1.8.3	Prior to induction, patient is reevaluated for anesthesia	___	___	___
_____	TX.2.3	Patient's physiological status is measured and assessed during anesthesia	___	___	___
_____	TX.5.4	Postoperative monitoring of patient includes:	___	___	___
_____	TX.5.4.1	- physiological and mental status	___	___	___
_____	TX.5.4.2	- pathological findings	___	___	___
_____	TX.5.4.3	- IVs, drugs, blood and components	___	___	___
_____	TX.5.4.4	- unusual events; postop complications and/or management	___	___	___
_____	TX.2.4.1	Patient discharge from the postanesthesia recovery area by licensed independent practitioner or by meeting Med Staff criteria	___	___	___
_____	IM.7.4.3.6	Name of licensed independent practitioner who discharged the patient from the anesthesia recovery area is recorded	___	___	___
_____	IM.7.4.3.4	Individual who provided nursing services in postop. anesthesia recovery area is identified	___	___	___

Operative Note

_____	IM.7.4.2	Operative note is documented immediately postop.	___	___	___
_____	IM.7.4.2	Operative note content includes (as applicable): - findings, procedures, specimen removed, postop. dx, name of surgeon and/or assistant	___	___	___
_____	IM.7.4.2.1	Operative note is authenticated by the surgeon	___	___	___
_____	IM.7.4.2.2	A progress note about the operation is entered immediately when there is a transcription delay	___	___	___

Special Populations:
Pediatric Record Includes

_____	PE.7.1	Developmental age, length or height, head circumference, weight	___	___	___
_____	PE.7.2	Education needs and daily activities	___	___	___
_____	PE.7.3	Immunization status	___	___	___
_____	PE.7.4	Family or guardian involvement expectations in assessment, treatment, continuing care of patient	___	___	___

Continued on next page

FIGURE 11 Closed Medical Record Form *(continued)*

Item #	Standard #		Y	N	NA
		Emergency Care			
____	IM.7.2.3	Care prior to arrival	___	___	___
____	IM.7.6.1.1	Time and means of arrival	___	___	___
____	IM.7.6.1.3	Conclusions at discharge: disposition, condition, instructions	___	___	___
____	IM.7.6.2	Copy of ED record to follow up provider	___	___	___
____	IM.7.6.2	- patient authorizes release of ED record	___	___	___
		Transfer not arbitrary	___	___	___
____	CC.6	- receiving hospital consents to transfer	___	___	___
____	CC.7	- information goes with patient	___	___	___
		Care of Dying Patient			
____	RI.1.2.8	Primary and secondary symptoms treated	___	___	___
____	RI.1.2.8	Pain management	___	___	___
____	RI.1.2.8	Psychological and spiritual concerns addressed	___	___	___
____	RI.1.2.6	MD orders for withholding resuscitative services	___	___	___
____	RI.1.2.7	or withdrawing life-sustaining treatment	___	___	___
		Ambulatory MR Includes:			
____	IM.7.5	- dx, conditions, procedures, drug allergies	___	___	___
____	IM.7.2.21	medications dispensed or prescribed	___	___	___
____	IM.7.5.1	- above list started by third visit	___	___	___
		Restraint and Seclusion			
____	TX.7.1	MD time-limited order	___	___	___
____	TX.7.1	Patient needs are attended	___	___	___
		Alleged/Suspected Abuse/Neglect			
____	PE.6.1	Assessment conducted with consent	___	___	___
____	PE.6.2	Safeguard evidence and/or information released by patient	___	___	___
____	PE.6.3	Legal notification, as required	___	___	___

The interview consists of two parts. During the first part, surveyors discuss the organization's quarterly medical record review processes and outcomes (IM.3.3.1). By the time this interview takes place, surveyors will have already assessed your organization's last four quarters of medical record reviews during the document review. Then surveyors might ask additional questions about your quarterly process for reviewing records.

FIGURE 12 Tally for Closed Medical Record Forms

Introduction
At the close of the Medical Record Interview, all of the completed Closed Medical Record forms are added up (totaled) by the hospital.
Please follow the instructions provided to complete the attached Tally.

Please Note:
The attached form, Tally for Closed Medical Record Forms, is **required to be used when tallying the forms.**

Instructions for Completing the Tally for Closed Medical Record Forms
1. Gather all the completed Closed Medical Record Forms.
2. Add up (total), **for EACH item:**
   a. the total number of forms with a **Y** entered for the item listed, then enter this number in *Column A*.
   b. the total number of forms with a **Y** or an **N** entered for item listed, then enter this number in *Column B*.

   Example:
   For the items "all medications prescribed and/or dispensed at discharge."
   three (3) forms have a Y;
   two (2) forms have an N;
   one (1) form has an NA.
   The total number of forms with a Y is three (3).
   Three (3) is entered into Column A.
   The total number of forms with a Y or an N is five (5).
   Five (5) is entered into Column B.
3. Complete Step 2 for all of the forms and items listed.
4. Complete Column C, for each item, by calculating the percentage of forms with a Y.
   To calculate the percentage:
   divide the number in Column A by the number in Column B.

   Example (as drawn from the example in step 2):
   Column A = 3
   Column B = 5
   3 divided by 5 = .60 = 60%
   Column C = 60

   Continued on next page

The Tally for Closed Medical Record Forms will also be completed by medical records staff and presented to surveyors during the medical record interview.

FIGURE 12 Tally for Closed Medical Record Forms *(continued)*

Instructions

1. Add up (total) all the Closed Medical Record Forms.
2. Enter, in Column A, the total number of forms with a Y entered for the item listed (see attached instructions for example).
3. Enter, in Column B, the total number of forms with a Y or an N entered for the items listed (see attached instructions for example).
4. Enter, in Column C, the percentage of forms with a Y (that is, divide the number in Column A by the number in Column B) (see attached instructions for example).

Item No.	Standard #		A #Y	B #Y and N	C A ÷ B = %
		General Items			
_____	IM.7.9	All entries in the record are dated and authenticated	___	___	___
_____	IM.7.2.1	Patient demographics includes name, address	___	___	___
		date of birth and legal representative (if applicable)	___	___	___
_____	IM.7.2.2	Legal status (for example, competency) documented	___	___	___
		for patients receiving mental health services	___	___	___
_____	RI.1.2.5	Patient involvement in formulation of advance directive is documented	___	___	___
_____	IM.7.2.10	Informed consent for treatment per policy (that is, risks, benefits, alternatives)	___	___	___
		Discharge Information			
_____	IM.7.3	Discharge summary or final progress note or transfer summary is present	___	___	___
_____	IM.7.2.21	Discharge information includes all meds prescribed or dispensed at discharge	___	___	___
_____	IM.7.3	reason patient was admitted	___	___	___
_____	IM.7.3	operative or invasive procedure reports	___	___	___
_____	IM.7.3	treatment rendered	___	___	___
_____	IM.7.3	discharge instructions	___	___	___
_____	IM.7.3	condition at discharge	___	___	___
_____	MS.6	Autopsy	___	___	___
		- met Medical Staff autopsy criteria	___	___	___
		History and Physical			
_____	PE.1.7.1	H and P completed within 24 hours of admission	___	___	___

FIGURE 12 Tally for Closed Medical Record Forms *(continued)*

Item No.	Standard #		A #Y	B #Y and N	C A ÷ B = %
_____	IM.7.2.6	Diagnosis and/or impression recorded on H and P			
_____	IM.7.2.7	Reason admitted is documented	___	___	___
_____	IM.7.2.8	Treatment plans documented in H and P	___	___	___
		Orders			
_____	IM.7.9	All orders are dated and authenticated	___	___	___
_____	IM.7.8.1	Verbal orders authenticated within organization's required time frame	___	___	___
_____	IM.7.9	House staff orders are countersigned	___	___	___
		Education			
		(patient and family, as applicable)			
_____	PF.2.1	Assessment of needs, abilities, and readiness	___	___	___
_____	PF.2.1.1	Assessment of cultural, religion, and limitations	___	___	___
_____	PF.2.2.1	Education about safe and effective use of meds	___	___	___
_____	PF.2.2.2	Education about safe and effective use of equipment	___	___	___
_____	PF.2.2.3	Education for diet, nutrition, drug or food interaction	___	___	___
_____	PF.2.2.4	Instructed about rehab techniques	___	___	___
_____	PF.2.2.5	Instructed about community resources	___	___	___
_____	PF.4.2	Educational process was interdisciplinary	___	___	___
_____	PF.2.2.6	Educated about when and how to obtain further care	___	___	___
_____	PF.3	Educated on discharge instructions	___	___	___
		Assessment of Patients			
_____	TX.3.4.1	Monitoring of meds' effect on the patient includes			
		assessment based on collective observations	___	___	___
		including the patient's own perception	___	___	___
_____	PE.1.1	Need for care or treatment, type of care and further			
		assessment is determined and documented	___	___	___
_____	PE.1.1	Physical, social, and psychologic assessments are documented	___	___	___
		Scope or intensity of further assessment is determined by:	___	___	___

Continued on next page

FIGURE 12 Tally for Closed Medical Record Forms *(continued)*

Item No.	Standard #		A #Y	B #Y and N	C A ÷ B = %
_____	PE.1.2.1	Patient diagnosis	____	____	____
_____	PE.1.2.2	Treatment setting	____	____	____
_____	PE.1.2.3	Patient desire for treatment	____	____	____
_____	PE.1.2.4	Patient response to previous treatment	____	____	____
_____	PE.1.3	Need for nutritional assessment is determined	____	____	____
_____	PE.1.4	Need for functional assessment is determined	____	____	____
_____	PE.1.6	Need for discharge planning is assessed	____	____	____
_____	TX.4.1	TPN requirement is based on assessment	____	____	____
_____	TX.4.2	Orders for TPN are based on assessment	____	____	____

Reassessment

Item No.	Standard #		A	B	C
_____	IM.7.2.15	Is present in the medical record	____	____	____
_____	PE.2.1	Is completed at specified times in the course of treatment	____	____	____
_____	PE.2.2	Is done to determine the patient's response to treatment	____	____	____
_____	PE.2.3	Is done when there is a significant change in the patient's condition	____	____	____
_____	PE.2.4	Is done when there is a significant change in the patient's diagnosis	____	____	____
_____	PE.3	Assessment data is integrated to identify and prioritize patient's needs for care and treatment	____	____	____
_____	PE.3.1	Care and treatment decisions are based on patient needs and/or priorities	____	____	____

Operative and Invasive Procedures

Item No.	Standard #		A	B	C
_____	PE.1.8	Preop H and P and diagnosis are recorded	____	____	____
_____	IM.7.4.1	- by licensed independent practitioner	____	____	____
_____	PE.1.8.1	Preanesthesia assessment (for example, risk, ASA) is documented	____	____	____
_____	TX.2.1	Preop plan for anesthesia is recorded	____	____	____
_____	PE.1.8.2	Patient determined to be appropriate anesthesia candidate	____	____	____
_____	PE.1.8.2.1	- by licensed independent practitioner	____	____	____
_____	TX.5.3.1	Nursing care plan recorded preop	____	____	____
_____	TX.5.3.2	A procedure/op plan is recorded preop	____	____	____

FIGURE 12 Tally for Closed Medical Record Forms *(continued)*

Item No.	Standard #		A #Y	B #Y and N	C A ÷ B = %
_____	PE.1.8.3	Prior to induction, patient is reevaluated for anesthesia	____	____	____
_____	TX.2.3	Patient physiological status measured and assessed during anesthesia	____	____	____
_____	TX.5.4	Post operative monitoring of patient includes:			
_____	TX.5.4.1	- physiological and mental status	____	____	____
_____	TX.5.4.2	- pathological findings	____	____	____
_____	TX.5.4.3	- IVs, drugs, blood and components	____	____	____
_____	TX.5.4.4	- unusual events; postop complications or management	____	____	____
_____	TX.2.4.1	Patient discharge from the postanesthesia recovery area by licensed independent practitioner	____	____	____
		or by meeting Med Staff criteria	____	____	____
_____	IM.7.4.3.6	Name of licensed independent practitioner who discharged the patient from the anesthesia recovery area is recorded	____	____	____
_____	IM.7.4.3.4	Individual who provided nursing services in postop anesthesia recovery area is identified	____	____	____

Operative Note

_____	IM.7.4.2	Operative note is documented immediately postop	____	____	____
_____	IM.7.4.2	Operative note content includes (as applicable):			
		- findings, procedures, specimen removed, postop dx, name of surgeon and/or assistant	____	____	____
_____	IM.7.4.2.1	Operative note is authenticated by the surgeon	____	____	____
_____	IM.7.4.2.2	A progress note about the operation is entered	____	____	____
		immediately when there is a transcription delay			

Special Populations
Pediatric Record Includes

_____	PE.7.1	Developmental age, length or height, head circumference, weight	____	____	____
_____	PE.7.2	Education needs and daily activities	____	____	____
_____	PE.7.3	Immunization status	____	____	____

Continued on next page

FIGURE 12 Tally for Closed Medical Record Forms *(continued)*

Item No.	Standard #		A #Y	B #Y and N	C A ÷ B = %
_____	PE.7.4	Family or guardian involvement expectations in assessment, treatment, continuing care of patient	_____	_____	_____
		Emergency Care			
_____	IM.7.2.3	Care prior to arrival	_____	_____	_____
_____	IM.7.6.1.1	Time and means of arrival	_____	_____	_____
_____	IM.7.6.1.3	Conclusions at discharge: disposition, condition, instructions	_____	_____	_____
_____	IM.7.6.2	Copy of ED record to follow-up provider	_____	_____	_____
_____	IM.7.6.2	- patient authorizes release of ED record transfer not arbitrary	_____	_____	_____
_____	CC.6	- receiving hospital consents to transfer	_____	_____	_____
_____	CC.7	- information goes with patient	_____	_____	_____
		Care of the Dying Patient			
_____	RI.1.2.8	Primary and secondary symptoms treated	_____	_____	_____
_____	RI.1.2.8	Pain management	_____	_____	_____
_____	RI.1.2.8	Psychological and spiritual concerns addressed	_____	_____	_____
_____	RI.1.2.6	MD orders for withholding resuscitative services	_____	_____	_____
_____	RI.1.2.7	or withdrawing life-sustaining treatment	_____	_____	_____
		Ambulatory MR Includes:			
_____	IM.7.5	- dx, conditions, procedures, drug allergies	_____	_____	_____
_____	IM.7.2.21	medications dispensed or prescribed	_____	_____	_____
_____	IM.7.5.1	- above list started by third visit	_____	_____	_____
		Restraint and Seclusion			
_____	TX.7.1	MD time-limited order	_____	_____	_____
_____	TX.7.1	Patient needs attending to	_____	_____	_____
		Alleged or Suspected Abuse or Neglect			
_____	PE.6.1	Assessment conducted with consent	_____	_____	_____
_____	PE.6.2	Safeguard evidence and/or info released by patient	_____	_____	_____
_____	PE.6.3	Legal notification, as required	_____	_____	_____

FIGURE 12 Tally for Closed Medical Record Forms *(continued)*

ORGANIZATION NAME   HOSPITAL ID NUMBER

CITY, STATE   FULL   FOC   CON FOLLOW-UP   SPL

MEDICAL RECORD STATISTICS (IM.7.7.2)

1. What is the average monthly patient discharge rate during the past 12 months? _____
2. What is the average number of operative procedures per month? _____
3. What is your organization's time frame for medical record delinquency, as specified in the medical staff rules and regulations? _____

   *If the medical staff has not defined a time frame, or if the time frame exceeds 30 days, the number of delinquent records should be based on 30 days after discharge. Do not count those records of patients discharged within the time frame.

4. For the start of survey and for each of the three quarters prior to survey, enter the total number of delinquent medical records *at that time* (as determined by the most recent count prior to that date):

	Start of survey	Three months prior	Six months prior	Nine months prior
Total delinq MR				

5. For each of the four quarters, how many of the delinquent medical records lack a history and physical examination (H&P)?

	Start of survey	Three months prior	Six months prior	Nine months prior
Lacking H and P				

6. For each of the four quarters, how many of the delinquent records lack an op report (if op report would be required)?

	Start of survey	Three months prior	Six months prior	Nine months prior
Lacking op report				

NOTE: A type I recommendation will be made for medical record delinquency if any of the following exist:
a. the average, over four quarters, of the total number of delinquent records exceeds 50% of the average monthly discharges (AMD); or
b. the average of the number of delinquent records lacking an H&P, based on at least four quarterly determinations, is fewer than nine, or 2% of the AMD, whichever is greater; or
c. the average of the number of delinquent records lacking an operative report, based on at least four quarterly determinations, is fewer than nine, or 2% of the average monthly operative procedures, whichever is greater.

Conditional accreditation will be recommended when the average, over four quarters, of the total number of delinquent records equals or exceeds twice the average monthly patient discharge rate.

NOTE: Medical record delinquency may be linked to an ineffective medical record review function (IM.3.3.1).

Director of Medical Records _____

                          Signature   (Please Print)   Date

Chief Executive Officer _____

                          Signature   (Please Print)   Date

FIGURE 13 Suggested Protocols for Request for Closed Medical Records

The following suggestions for the request for closed medical records *do not* preclude the survey team from adding criteria (for example, specification of time frame, patient gender or age).

PART I: Types of Records/Topics

Discharge Disposition
home with ventilator
home with TPN expired with autopsy

Emergency Services
treated and released patients (not admitted as an inpatient)
victims of suspected or alleged abuse
transfer from ED to another facility

Medical
CHF
MI or AMI
ICU or special care unit
diabetes ketoacidosis
terminally ill patient (for example, carcinoma with advanced metastases; care of the dying patient)

DNR order
life support withdrawn
referred to Ethics Committee

Obstetrics/ Newborn
C-section with infant record
vaginal delivery, epidural, with infant record

Outpatient/ Ambulatory Care
surgical or endoscopic procedure with IV sedation
clinics available at this site
house staff

Pediatrics
asthma diagnosis
gastroenteritis diagnosis

Psychiatry
restraint, seclusion and/or psychosurgery,
depression or major depression diagnosis
dual diagnoses (for example, substance abuse and depression)
medical detoxification
ECT

Selection criteria to be used in designating closed medical records to be examined for the medical record interview

FIGURE 13 Suggested Protocols for Request for Closed Medical Records *(continued)*

Surgery   cholecystectomy (may also be an outpatient laproscopic procedure)
joint replacement
cardiac catheterization
PTCA with or without CABG
surgical procedure for carcinoma with (advanced) metastases
DNR order
life support withdrawal order
referred to Ethics committee

Other Specialties/ Disciplines   Podiatric
Dental
Physical Rehabilitation

PART 2: *Number of Records*

Number of Operating Beds	Number of Records Suggested
10	8
20	13
30	17
50	23
100	29
150	32
200	34
250	35
300	36
400	37
500–600	38
700–1000	39
1500 +	40

The second part of the interview deals with IM.7 and related standards. The surveyors will review the closed medical forms with staff members who completed the forms and verify the findings with a sample of the record(s). By this time, surveyors will have reviewed open records during patient care setting visits. The results of the closed medical record review will be merged with those from the reviews of open records, as appropriate.

Resource Center Visit

To assess the availability of knowledge-based resources in the organization, the administrator will pay a visit to your organization's resource center or library. The surveyor will want to talk with the manager of the resource center or librarian. Other staff may also participate, at the discretion of your organization. The administrator surveyor will ask about how your organization's needs for knowledge-based information were assessed. Staff should also be prepared to talk about and demonstrate the various processes you have in place for identifying, organizing, retrieving, analyzing, and delivering knowledge-based information. The surveyor will be interested in how these processes are linked with the organization's internal information systems and with appropriate external database(s) and information networks.

Feedback Activities

Surveyors will continually communicate survey findings to the organization. A short daily briefing for key leaders will be given each morning of the survey, except on the first day. Surveyors will provide leaders with their general reactions to the previous day's activities and point out any patterns of significant concern they may have identified. This is also a time for surveyors to request any missing information or to make necessary adjustments to the survey schedule. On the last day of the survey, the survey team then conducts an exit conference with your organization's leaders. The surveyors should be able to provide a reasonable, accurate summary of findings on completion of the survey.

Post-Survey Activities

After the on-site survey, your organization's survey findings are analyzed and aggregated at the Joint Commission. These results are reviewed internally by professional staff, and decision rules are then applied to reach an accreditation decision and define any necessary follow-up requirements. Then, if your organization's accreditation decision falls within established parameters, you are directly notified of your accreditation decision. Accreditation findings that raise specific issues are reviewed by the Joint Commission's Accreditation Committee, which then reaches a final decision.*

■ Conclusion

This chapter has presented your organization with an overview of the new survey process and, more specifically, how the management of information function will be surveyed. It is important, however, to remember that the management of information is an organizationwide function. Data and information is an integral component in the performance of every other function identified in the *AMH*. Therefore, as surveyors assess other key functions (for example, care of patients or managing the environment of care), they will also observe how well your management of information processes are being performed.

---

*Readers interested in learning more about the accreditation and decision process can obtain copies of *Making Accreditation Decisions* from the Joint Commission by calling 708/916-5800.

APPENDIX A

The "Management of Information" Chapter from the 1995 *CAMH*

■ An Overview of the *CAMH* Chapter

This appendix contains the direct citation of the "Management of Information" chapter from the 1995 *Comprehensive Accreditation Manual for Hospitals (CAMH)*, and provides comprehensive standards-related information concerning the management of information function. It includes the standards, scoring guidelines, and aggregation information (aggregation rules, accreditation decision grid). This information should help you understand Joint Commission requirements as well as assist you in conducting self-assessment activities.

The *CAMH* chapter begins with a **preamble.** The preamble describes the function upon which the chapter focuses and explains its significance, rationale, theoretical underpinnings, and relationship to other functions. The preamble also describes the goal and scope of the function and the processes involved in achieving the goal. Definitions of key terms appear on the page with the first use of the term.

The management of information function is illustrated in a flowchart (Figure 14, page 165, and Figure 1, page 12) that depicts the processes in the function and indicates how the standards are organized in the chapter. The function is then explained in an example of a practical application. This application shows how the management of information function would apply in the hospital treatment of a 4-year-old girl injured in an automobile accident—a scenario depicted throughout the *CAMH*.

Once the function and its processes are explained, the standards are presented (see Exhibits 1 and 2, pages 166–167). Here, expectations that must be met for accreditation purposes are set forth. Management of information standards are identified by the chapter acronym—IM—and the number of the standard. Scoring guidelines follow while scoring scales appear in the margin opposite the standards. The scoring scale can be used to capture the score you assign to a standard during any type of self-assessment you choose to perform. It contains six rankings—the numbers 1 through 5 and NA (not applicable). These rankings reflect the following levels of compliance:

SCORE 1 **Substantial compliance** indicates that the organization consistently meets all major provisions of the standard (some provisions may be in the intent).

SCORE 2 **Significant compliance** indicates that the organization meets most provisions of the standard.

SCORE 3 **Partial compliance** indicates that the organization meets some provisions of the standard.

SCORE 4 **Minimal compliance** indicates that the organization meets few provisions of the standard.

SCORE 5 **Noncompliance** indicates that the organization fails to meet the provisions of the standard.

NA **Not applicable** indicates that the standard does not apply to the organization.

FIGURE 14 Management of Information Function

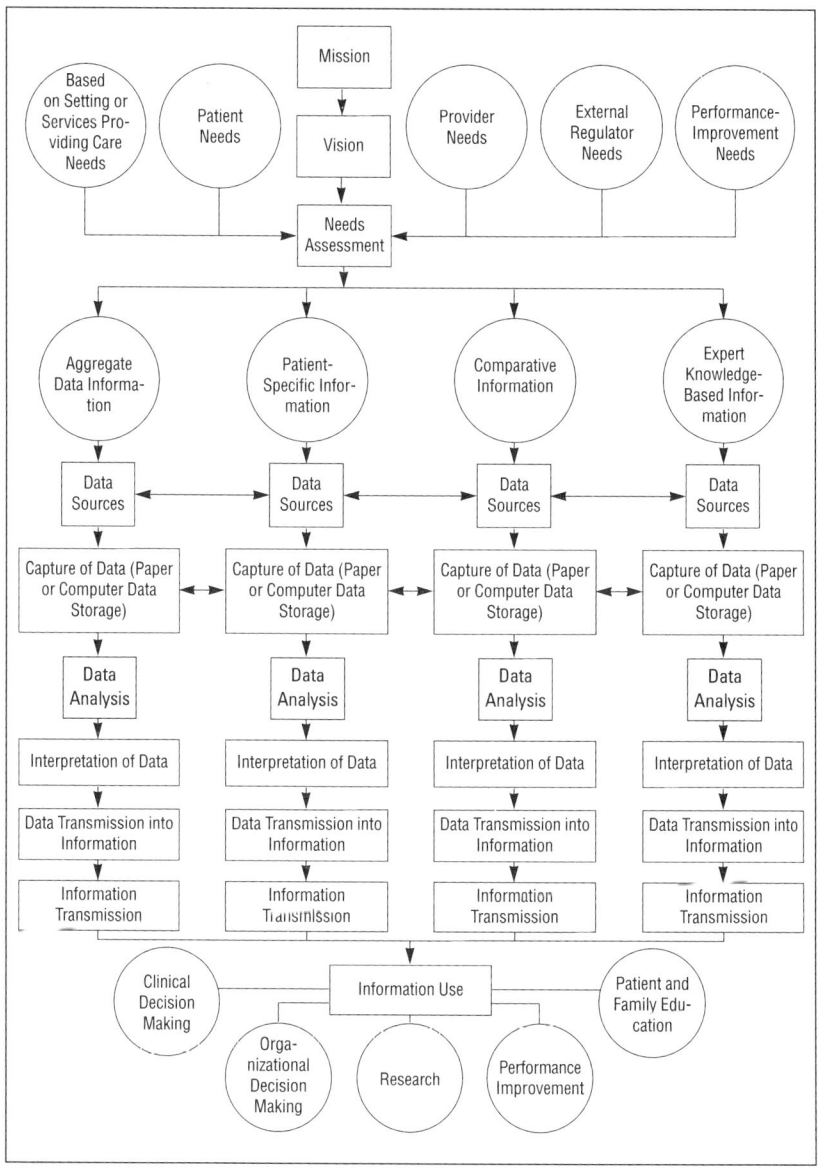

This flowchart graphically represents most of the important activities and processes, particularly the risk points, in the management of information function.

EXHIBIT 1 A Typical Section from a Functional Chapter of the 1995 *CAMH*

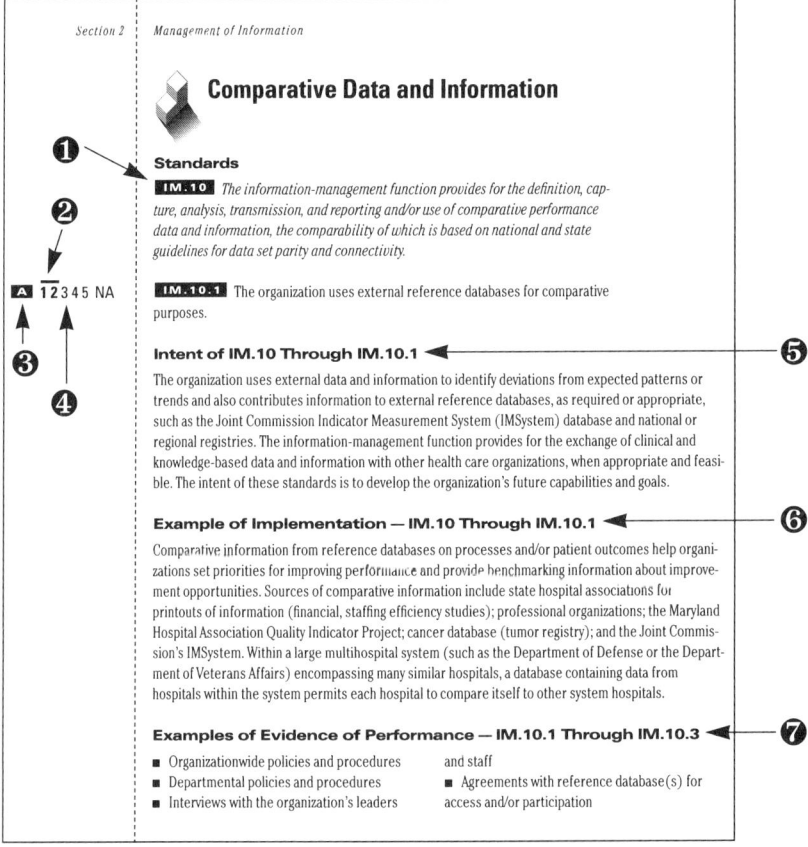

❶ **Standard**—States expectations that must be met for accreditation purposes

❷ **Cap**—Defines the maximum impact the score of a standard can have on the grid element score

❸ **Alphabetic Set Designation**—Indicates the set to which a standard belongs in aggregation

❹ **Scoring Scale**—Reflects the five possible levels of standards compliance

❺ **Intent Statement**—Explains the rationale, meaning, and significance of the standard(s)

❻ **Example of Implementation**—Outlines strategies, activities, and/or processes that can be used to meet the intent of a standard(s)

❼ **Examples of Evidence of Performance**—Provides insight into the sources a surveyor may seek or you may present as evidence that your organization complies with a standard(s)

Appendix A   The 1995 *CAMH* Excerpt

EXHIBIT 2 An Example Page from the *CAMH* Providing Scoring Information and Aggregation Summary

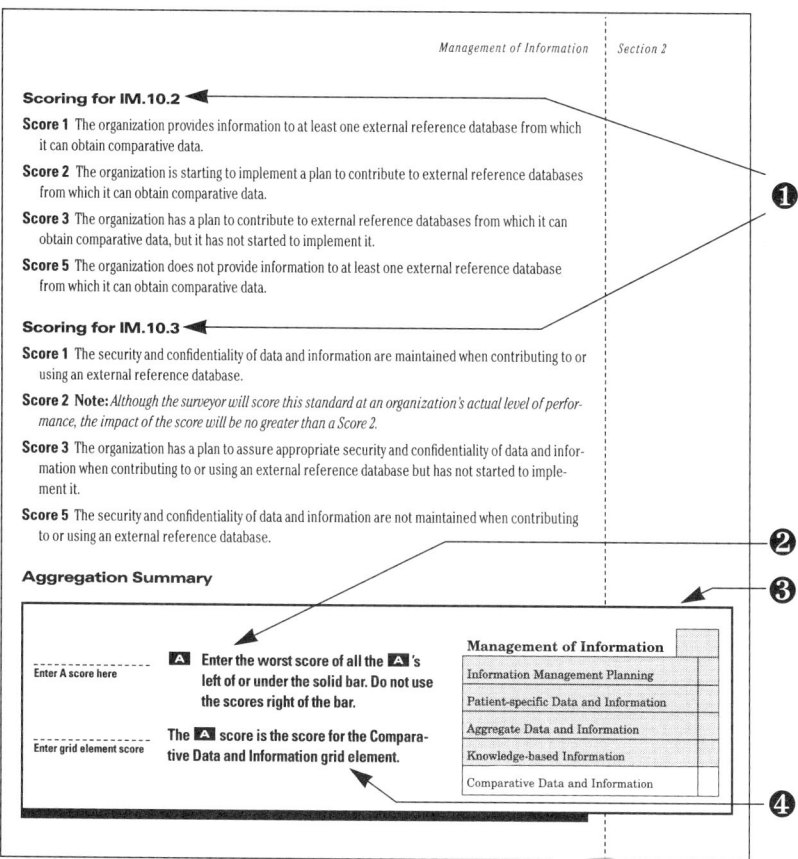

❶ **Scoring**—Identifies the levels of compliance with a standard(s); can be expressed quantitatively or qualitatively

❷ **Directions for Determining a Set Score**

❸ **Aggregation Summary**—Contains directions for determining the set score(s) from the individual scores assigned to standards in a grid element and also for determining the grid element score from the set score(s)

❹ **Directions for Determining the Grid Element Score**

Aggregation is essentially the process used by the Joint Commission to consolidate scores for individual standards into an organization's accreditation decision. It involves the use of several tools, including aggregation rules and the accreditation decision grid (see Exhibit 3, page 169). During aggregation, the scores for all the standards in the management of information function are aggregated into the five performance areas or grid elements: information-management planning, patient-specific data and information, aggregate data and information, knowledge-based information, and comparative data and information. These correlate with the sections of the management of information standards. Then, each of these scores is aggregated into one score for the management of information function.

Aggregation information is found in two places around the scoring scale. An **alphabetic character** appears to the left of the scale. This alphabetic character designates the set to which the standard belongs. A solid bar appears over the scoring scale of many standards. (In this book, a screened box replaces the bar used in the manuals.) This bar stops at a specific number on the scale and is used to indicate the **cap** assigned to the standard. The score at which the standard is capped appears in boldfaced type. Any standard that does not aggregate to the grid element in which it appears is typeset in italics. An explanatory note accompanies many of these standards. Aggregation information is explained in the "Accreditation Decision Process" chapter of the *CAMH*.

The **Intent** statement explains the rationale, meaning, and significance of the standard. The standard's purpose is clearly stated with any additional relevant information regarding the standard. During an accreditation survey, organizations must demonstrate that they meet the intent of the standard.

Strategies, activities, and/or processes that an organization may use to meet the standards are outlined in the **Examples of Implementation.** Each example is adapted and condensed from activities carried out in actual health care organizations. The examples are not intended to represent all the implementation

Appendix A The 1995 *CAMH* Excerpt

EXHIBIT 3 The 1995 Hospital Accreditation Services Accreditation Decision Grid

```
                        JCAHO
              Hospital Accreditation Services
               Accreditation Decision Grid
```

Organization: Your Hospital   Survey Date: 1/1/95
Location: Anywhere, USA

PATIENT-FOCUSED FUNCTIONS	ORGANIZATIONAL FUNCTIONS	ORGANIZATIONAL FUNCTIONS CONTINUED
Patient Rights and Organizational Ethics	**Improving Organizational Performance**	**Management of Information**
Patient Rights	Plan	Information Management Planning
Organizational Ethics	Design	Patient-specific Data and Information
	Measure	Aggregate Data and Information
Assessment of Patients	Assess	Knowledge-based Information
Initial Assessment	Improve	Comparative Data and Information
Pathology and Clinical Laboratory Services–Waived Testing		**Surveillance, Prevention, and Control of Infection**
Reassessment	**Leadership**	
Care Decisions	Organizational Planning	Surveillance, Prevention, and Control of Infection
Structures Supporting the Assessment of Patients	Directing Departments	
	Integrating Services	**STRUCTURES WITH FUNCTIONS**
Additional Requirements for Specific Patient Populations	Role in Improving Performance	
	Management of the Environment of Care	**Governance**
Care of Patients	Design	Governance
Planning and Providing Care	Implementation	
Anesthesia Care	Measurement Systems	**Management**
Medication Use	Social Environment	Management
Nutrition Care	**Management of Human Resources**	
Operative and Other Invasive Procedures	Human Resources Planning	**Medical Staff**
Rehabilitation Care and Services	Orientation, Training, and Education of Staff	Organization, Bylaws, Rules and Regulations
Special Treatment Procedures	Competence Assessment	Credentialing
Education	Staff Rights Mechanisms	**Nursing**
Patient and Family Education and Responsibilities		Nursing
	1 = Substantial Compliance 2 = Significant Compliance 3 = Partial Compliance 4 = Minimal Compliance 5 = No Compliance N = Not Applicable P = Defer to Primary Service	**Special Type I Recommendation(s)**
Continuum of Care		
Continuum of Care		

1995 HAS Grid - Effective: January, 1995   ©1994

strategies that have the potential to meet the intent of a standard or group of standards. You are encouraged to be innovative in your approach to meeting the intent of the standards.

Examples of Evidence of Performance provide insight into sources from which a surveyor may seek evidence or that you may present to a surveyor to show that your organization complies with the intent of a standard(s). Such sources can include any organizational or departmental documents; interviews with leaders, staff, patients, and families; patient unit visits; and medical record review. The examples of evidence of performance are intended to help you determine which evidence will most accurately and clearly indicate your organization's level of performance in meeting the intent of the standard, and to provide insight into the relationship between the standards and the survey process. They are not intended to represent all possible forms and sources of evidence. If you choose to implement an innovative approach to comply with a standard(s), you should plan from the beginning the evidence of performance that you would provide to a surveyor to demonstrate compliance.

The **Aggregation Summary** (see Exhibit 4, below) contains directions for consolidating the individual scores assigned to the standard in a grid element. The aggregation summary appears in a box immediately following the last set of scoring in each grid element within the chapter. (Aggregation and how to aggregate the individual scores you assign to the standards are explained in detail in the "Accreditation Decision Process" chapter of the *CAMH*.) Once a grid element score has been determined, the score can be transferred to the accreditation decision grid (see Exhibit 3). Once the accreditation decision is scored, the decision rules are applied to determine an accreditation decision and any necessary follow-up monitoring. (These are found in Appendix E of the *CAMH*.)

EXHIBIT 4 Aggregation Summary

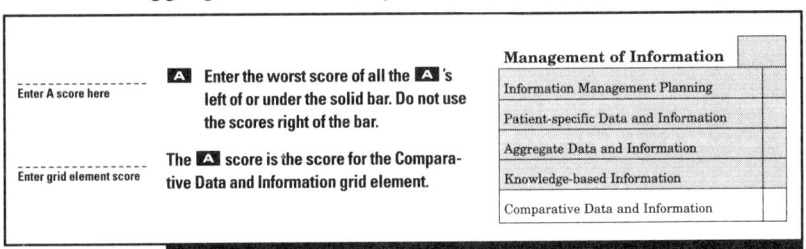

An example of an aggregation summary, which contains directions for consolidating the individual scores assigned to the standard in a grid element.

The *CAMH* "Management of Information" Chapter

■ Preamble

An organization's provision of health care is a complex endeavor that is highly dependent on information.* This includes information about the science of care, the individual patient, the care provided, the results of care, and the performance of the organization itself. Furthermore, because many individuals and departments** within the organization provide care, their work must be coordinated and integrated. Because of this dependence on information and the need to coordinate and integrate services, health care organizations must treat information as an important resource to be managed effectively and efficiently. Managing information is an active, planned activity. The organization's leaders have overall responsibility for this activity—just as they do for managing the organization's human, material, and financial resources.

---

* **Information** An interpreted set(s) of data; organized data that provide a basis for decision making.

** A **department** is defined in the *CAMH* as any structural unit of the health care organization, whether it is called a department, a service, a unit, or something similar.

Information management is a function*—a set of processes and activities—focused on meeting the organization's information needs. Its goal is to obtain, manage, and use information to enhance and improve individual and organizational performance in patient care, governance, management, and support processes. Although the efficiency and effectiveness of information-management processes may be affected by the technologies employed (for example, computerization), the principles of good information management (as reflected in these standards) are relevant regardless of the technology used. Therefore, although these standards are compatible with current, cutting-edge technologies (and, it is hoped, with future technologies), they are intended to be equally applicable in organizations that are not computerized.

These standards describe a vision of effective and continuously improving information management in health care organizations. The objectives related to achieving this vision are

- more timely and easy access to complete information throughout the organization;
- improved data** accuracy;
- demonstrated balance of proper levels of security† versus ease of access;
- use of aggregate‡ data, along with external knowledge databases and comparative data, to pursue opportunities for improvement;
- redesign of important information-related processes to improve efficiency; and
- greater collaboration and information sharing to enhance patient care.

For most organizations, achieving all of these objectives will require varying periods of time of up to five years. Thus, the scoring guidelines for this chapter will accommodate the time

---

* **function** A group of activities and processes with a common goal.
** **data** Uninterrupted observations or facts.
† **security** The protection of data from intentional or unintentional destruction, modification, or disclosure.
‡ **aggregate** To combine standardized data and information.

needed for this transition to implement effective organization-wide information management.

The standards focus on the key information-management processes of organizationwide planning to meet internal and external information needs. The standards also focus on managing patient-specific data and information, aggregate data and information, expert knowledge-based information*, and comparative performance data and information. Specifically, the standards address

- identification of the organization's information needs;
- structural design of the information-management system;
- definition and capture** of data and information;
- data analysis and transformation† of data into information;
- transmission‡ and reporting of data and information; and
- assimilation and use of information.

The organization's leaders have important roles and responsibilities if an organizationwide approach to information management is to be achieved, maintained, and improved. Also, staff at many levels must be educated and trained in managing and using information.

The performance-improvement framework in the "Improving Organizational Performance" chapter of the *CAMH* is used to design, measure, assess, and improve the organization's performance of the information-management function.

The terms used in this chapter are defined as they are used in the context of the organizational function and may not reflect common dictionary usage.

---

* **knowledge-based information** A collection of stored facts, models, and information that can be used for designing and redesigning processes and for problem solving. In the context of the *CAMH*, knowledge-based information is found in the clinical, scientific, and management literature.

** **capture** The acquisition or recording of data and information.

† **transformation** The process of changing the form of data representation (for example, changing data into information using decision analysis tools).

‡ **transmission** The sending of data and information from one location to another.

■ Practical Application

Four years ago, during routine staffing studies done as part of the internal needs assessment prior to budget planning, the leaders of the aforementioned hospital determined that an average of 31% of the time available to patient care staff was spent documenting patient care activities. [Editor's Note: This hospital is part of the scenario depicted in the *CAMH*.] Based on national initiatives recently published in the Institute of Medicine's *Healthy People 2000 Report*, and on further investigation and study, the hospital governing board approved a large capital fundraising plan to provide a computer-based patient record.

After various prototypes were assessed, the hospital's leaders chose software packages to support all their defined information-management needs. They then selected appropriate hardware to run the programs. The total system includes a series of bedside terminals in all patient care areas, including the pediatric intensive care unit (PICU) that permits all patient care staff to chart their assessment, care, and treatment activities without leaving the patient's side. In addition, all laboratory and radiology reports are now transmitted electronically to each patient's file.

The software not only supports the hospital's business functions, but also permits the aggregation of patient-specific data with other types of aggregate-data-management activities, such as each patient's medication profile. In moving from a traditional hospital library to a resource center, the hospital added on-line modem capability to query the major health care literature databases. Infection control statistics are calculated on the system, with charts generated for reporting of rates and trends to key infection-control staff. Staff conduct clinical research at this hospital, and medication trials are documented in computer files. Also, the hospital both contributes to and receives reports from several external databases for performance comparison.

See also the flowcharts or process diagrams for "Leadership," "Management of the Environment of Care," "Management of Human Resources," "Surveillance, Prevention and Control of Infection," and "Improving Organizational Performance" and the chapters in Section 1 of the *CAMH*.

Information Management Planning

■ Standard

IM.1

A 1 2 3 4 5 NA   Information-management processes are planned and designed to meet the health care organization's internal and external information needs.

■ Intent of IM.1

The organization assesses its needs for information management based on its mission, goals, services, personnel, mode(s) of service delivery (for example, hospital, home care, ambulatory), resources, and access to affordable technology. A comprehensive assessment of needs considers, as appropriate,

- the organization's type, structure, size, and complexity;
- the individuals and groups whom the function is serving or will serve (for example, governance, managers, clinical staff, inpatients and ambulatory patients, patients' families, payers and purchasers, regulatory bodies, accrediting bodies);
- the support needed for planning purposes;
- the support needed for education services and any research activity;
- any national and state guidelines for data set parity* and connectivity** in interfacing information systems;
- the requirements for internal and external transmission of data and information;
- longitudinal data and information reporting needs;

---

* **data parity** The equivalency of data.
** **data connectivity** The ability to link data.

- the requirements for internally and externally generated data and information to support continuous improvement in performance;
- the requirements for comparing the organization's performance with internal past performance, with that of other organizations (benchmarking), and with information from the literature (for example, practice guidelines);
- the appropriateness of various technologies;
- the costs of various technologies;
- the need to support customer and supplier relationships;
- the analysis of resource use for patients with particular clinical problems to enhance the cost-effectiveness of care;
- the enhancement of work flow activity;
- the support needed for clinical and administrative decision making; and
- the direction (for example, of library services, medical records, computer services) needed for the scope and complexity of services provided.

■ Examples of Evidence of Performance — IM.1
- A written plan for information management that is either independent or part of the overall organizational plans
- Meeting minutes
- Reports

■ Scoring for IM.1

SCORE 1 Information-management processes are based on a comprehensive assessment of needs that considers, when appropriate, the elements listed in the intent.

SCORE 2 With a few, minor exceptions, information-management processes are based on a comprehensive assessment of needs that considers, when appropriate, the elements listed in the intent.

SCORE 3 Information-management processes are based on an assessment of needs, but the assessment does

Appendix A   The 1995 *CAMH* Excerpt   **177**

not consider, when appropriate, a significant number of the elements listed in the intent.

SCORE 4   Information-management processes are based on an assessment of needs, but the assessment considers only a few of the elements listed in the intent.

SCORE 5   Information-management processes are not based on a comprehensive assessment of needs.

▰ Standards

IM.1.1

A 1 2 3 4 5 NA   The information-management processes within and among organization departments, the medical staff, the administration, and the governing body and with outside services and agencies are appropriate for the organization's size and complexity.

IM.1.1.1

A 1 2 3 4 5 NA   Direction, staffing, and material resource allocations are based on the organization's scope and complexity of services provided.

IM.1.1.2

A 1 2 3 4 5 NA   Based on the organization's information needs, appropriate staff participate in assessing, selecting, and integrating health care information technology and, as appropriate, using efficient interactive information-management systems for clinical and organizational information.

▰ Intent of IM.1.1 Through IM.1.1.2

Health care organizations vary in size, complexity, governance, structure, and decision needs. The information-management processes used are based on an analysis of the entire organization and depend on staff input in a variety of areas and services. Appropriate individuals ensure that required data and information are provided for patient care, research, education, and management at every level of the organization.

■ Examples of Evidence of Performance—IM.1.1 Through IM.1.1.2

- Planning documents
- Interviews with appropriate staff
- Observations
- Meeting minutes

■ Scoring for IM.1.1

SCORE 1 Evidence indicates that internal and external information-management processes are appropriate for the organization's size and complexity.

SCORE 2 Evidence indicates that, with a few, minor exceptions, internal and external information-management processes are appropriate for the organization's size and complexity.

SCORE 3 Evidence indicates that some internal information-management processes are not appropriate for the organization's size and complexity.
OR
Evidence indicates that some external information-management processes are not appropriate for the organization's size and complexity.

SCORE 4 Evidence indicates that only a few internal information-management processes are appropriate for the organization's size and complexity.
OR
Evidence indicates that none of the external information-management processes is appropriate for the organization's size and complexity.

SCORE 5 Evidence indicates that none of the internal and external information-management processes is appropriate for the organization's size and complexity.

■ Scoring for IM.1.1.1

SCORE 1 Evidence indicates that the organization provides direction, staffing, and material resource allocations based on its scope and complexity of services.

SCORE 2 Evidence indicates that, with a few, minor exceptions, the organization provides direction, staffing, and material resource allocations based on its scope and complexity of services.

SCORE 3 Evidence indicates that the organization does not consistently provide direction, staffing, and material resource allocations based on its scope and complexity of services.

SCORE 4 Evidence indicates that the organization seldom provides direction, staffing, and material resource allocations based on its scope and complexity of services.

SCORE 5 Evidence indicates that the organization does not provide direction, staffing, and material resource allocations based on its scope and complexity of services.

■ Scoring for IM.1.1.2

SCORE 1 Evidence indicates that appropriate staff participate in assessing, selecting, and integrating health care information technology and, as appropriate, using efficient interactive information-management systems for clinical and organizational information.

SCORE 2 Evidence indicates that, with a few, minor exceptions, appropriate staff participate in assessing, selecting, and integrating health care information technology and, as appropriate, using efficient interactive information-management systems for clinical and organizational information.

SCORE 3 Evidence indicates that appropriate staff do not consistently participate in assessing, selecting, and integrating health care information technology and, as appropriate, using efficient interactive information-management systems for clinical and organizational information.

SCORE 4 Evidence indicates that appropriate staff seldom participate in assessing, selecting, and integrating health care information technology and, as appropriate, using efficient interactive information-management systems for clinical and organizational information.

SCORE 5 Evidence indicates that appropriate staff do no participate in assessing, selecting, and integrating health care information technology and, as appropriate, using efficient interactive information-management systems for clinical and organizational information.

Standards

IM.2 *The information-management function provides for information confidentiality*, security, and integrity**.*

IM.2.1

A 1 2 3 4 5 NA The organization determines the need for and appropriate levels of security and confidentiality of data and information.

---

* **confidentiality** The safekeeping of data and information as restricted to individuals who have need, reason, and permission for access to such data and information.

** **integrity** The accuracy, consistency, and completeness of data.

Appendix A   The 1995 *CAMH* Excerpt

IM.2.2
A 1 2 3 4 5 NA   The organization determines how data and information can be retrieved on a timely and easy basis without compromising the data's and information's security and confidentiality.

IM.2.2.1
A 1 2 3 4 5 NA   A written organizational and medical staff policy requires that medical records may be removed from the organization's jurisdiction and safekeeping only in accordance with a court order, subpoena, or statute.

IM.2.2.2
A 1 2 3 4 5 NA   The organization has a functioning mechanism designed to preserve the confidentiality of data and information identified as sensitive or requiring extraordinary means to protect patient privacy.

IM.2.3
A 1 2 3 4 5 NA   The organization has a functioning mechanism designed to safeguard records and information against loss, destruction, tampering, and unauthorized access or use.

■ Intent of IM.2 Through IM.2.3

The organization is responsible for maintaining the security and confidentiality of data and information. The conflict between data sharing and data confidentiality is addressed. The organization determines the level of security and/or confidentiality for different categories of information. Access to each information category is appropriate to the user's title and job function. An effective process identifies at least
- the individual having access to information;
- the information to which an individual has access;

- the obligation of the individual who has access to information to keep it confidential;
- the release of health information and/or removal of the medical record; and
- the mechanism designed to secure information against unauthorized intrusion, corruption, and damage.

■ Examples of Implementation—IM.2 Through IM.2.3

1. When certain portions of the medical record are so confidential that extraordinary means are necessary to preserve their privacy (such as in the treatment of some psychiatric disorders), these portions may be stored separately, provided that the complete record is readily available when required for current medical care or follow-up, review functions, or performance-improvement activities.
2. Access to computer files can be controlled through security codes or by restricting certain operations to particular terminals. For instance, the computer terminals in the finance department can be accessed only by individuals in that department and only to perform financial transactions.
3. An example of security planning is a disaster recovery plan that addresses such items as theft, vandalism, loss of critical data, provision of emergency power, and fire and flood recovery.
4. When an organization is in transition from manual methods to computerization or from one type of computer system to another (for example, mainframe to local area networks), it needs to consider security carefully. For instance, backup provisions are in place as critical applications are being moved to different environments.

■ Examples of Evidence of Performance— IM.2.1 Through IM.2.3

- Organizationwide policies and procedures
- Departmental policies and procedures
- Protocols

- Interviews with appropriate staff
- Observations

■ Scoring for IM.2

This standard is not scored.

■ Scoring for IM.2.1

SCORE 1   The organization has a process(es) in place designed to ensure sufficient security and confidentiality for its data and information. The process(es) addresses at least the five items listed in the intent.

AND

The organization has a plan in place that addresses the five items listed in the intent for any new data and information collection, storage, and retrieval system(s) that may be implemented.

SCORE 2   The organization has a process(es) in place designed to ensure sufficient security and confidentiality for its data and information. The process(es) addresses four of the five items listed in the intent.

SCORE 3   The organization has a process(es) in place designed to ensure sufficient security and confidentiality for its data and information. The process(es) addresses three of the five items listed in the intent.

OR

The organization does not have a plan in place that addresses any of the five items listed in the intent for any new data and information collection, storage, and retrieval system(s) that may be implemented.

SCORE 4   The organization has a process(es) in place designed to ensure sufficient security and confidentiality for its data and information. The process(es) addresses fewer than three of the five items listed in the intent.

SCORE 5 The organization does not have a process in place designed to ensure sufficient security and confidentiality for its data and information.

■ Scoring for IM.2.2

SCORE 1 The organization has systems in place for timely and easy access to data and information, and the data and information are safeguarded.

SCORE 2 The organization has systems in place for timely and easy access to data and information. However, not all data and information are safeguarded.

SCORE 3 The organization has systems in place for timely and easy access to data and information. However, there is only a plan to safeguard the data and information, and the plan is not implemented.

SCORE 4 The organization has systems in place for timely and easy access to data and information. However, evidence indicates that these systems are ineffective, and the data and information are not safeguarded.

SCORE 5 The organization does not have systems in place for timely and easy access to data and information, and the data and information are not safeguarded.

■ Scoring for IM.2.2.1

SCORE 1 The organization has a written organizational and medical staff policy requiring that medical records may be removed from the organization's jurisdiction and safekeeping only in accordance with a court order, subpoena, or statute.
AND
This policy is enforced.

SCORE 5 The organization does not have a written organizational and medical staff policy requiring that medical records may be removed from the organization's jurisdiction and safekeeping only in accordance with a court order, subpoena, or statute.

OR

If the organization has such a policy, it is not enforced.

■ Scoring for IM.2.2.2

SCORE 1 Evidence indicates that the organization has a functioning mechanism designed to preserve the confidentiality of data and information identified as sensitive or requiring extraordinary means to protect patient privacy.

SCORE 3 Evidence indicates that the organization has a functioning mechanism designed to preserve the confidentiality of data and information identified as sensitive or requiring extraordinary means to protect patient privacy; however, it is not consistently enforced.

SCORE 5 Evidence indicates that the organization does not have a functioning mechanism designed to preserve the confidentiality of data and information identified as sensitive or requiring extraordinary means to protect patient privacy.

■ Scoring for IM.2.3

SCORE 1 Evidence indicates that records and information are protected against loss, destruction, tampering, and unauthorized access or use.

SCORE 3 Evidence indicates that not all records and information are protected against loss, destruction, tampering, and unauthorized access or use.

SCORE 5 Evidence indicates that records and information are not protected at all times against loss, destruction, tampering, and unauthorized access or use.

■ Standards

IM.3 *When feasible, uniform data definitions* and methods for capturing data are in place.*

IM.3.1
A 1 2 3 4 5 NA Whenever possible, minimum data sets**, data definitions, codes, classifications, and terminology are standardized throughout the organization.

IM.3.1.1
A 1 2 3 4 5 NA The organization references externally standardized sets, definitions, codes, classifications, and terminology (when available) when developing its organization standards.

IM.3.2
A 1 2 3 4 5 NA The organization collects data in a timely, economical, and efficient manner and with the degree of accuracy, completeness, and discrimination necessary for their intended use.

IM.3.3
A 1 2 3 4 5 NA The organization implements mechanisms designed to ascertain that bias† in the data is minimized and to assess the data's reliability, validity‡, and accuracy on an ongoing basis.

■ Intent of IM.3 Through IM.3.3

To facilitate comparison of data and information within and among organizations, terminology, definitions, vocabulary,

---

* **data definition** The identification of the data to be used in analysis.
** **minimum data sets** An agreed-on and accepted set of terms and definitions constituting a core of data; a collection of related data items.
† **bias** An effect tending to produce results that depart systematically from the true value (to be distinguished from random error).
‡ **validity** Verification of correctness.

and nomenclature are standardized whenever possible. Standardization also includes abbreviations and symbols. When standardizing terminology, the organization considers national and state guidelines for data set uniformity and connectivity, as available. Uniformly applied and accepted data definitions, codes, classifications, and terminology support data aggregation and analysis and provide criteria for decision analysis. Quality control systems are in place to monitor data content and collection, and are designed to ensure timely and economical collection of data. The health care team collecting and reviewing the data is responsible for information accuracy and completeness.

■ Examples of Implementation—IM.3 Through IM.3.3

1. Standardized coding and reporting systems include public health reporting requirements; coding systems for discharge diagnoses for billing; coding of procedures; reporting to state and federal health planning and analysis agencies; internal use for case mix analysis; and data for performance improvement activities. Some coding systems include International Classification of Disease—9th Revision—Clinical Modification (ICD-9-CM), Systematized Nomenclature of Pathology (SNOP), Systematized Nomenclature of Medicine (SNOMED), and Current Procedural Terminology (CPT). Some standardized nursing nomenclatures include the North American Nursing Diagnoses Association List of Approved Diagnoses, the Nursing Interventions Classification from the University of Iowa, and the Omaha System for Community and Ambulatory Care. Quality control examples include defining criteria for data capture, data input, or recording; defining statistically appropriate sampling procedures; reviewing medical records for completeness, accuracy, and timeliness; and reviewing and addressing the qualifications of persons responsible for performing the quality measurement. Another quality control example is single data entry with multiple uses and a defined process for checking data.

Library control examples include the need for uniformity in the organization and retrieval of knowledge-based information. Uniform reporting is essential for participation in interlibrary networks. Tools used to assure uniformity include Medical Subject Headings (MESH), the National Library of Medicine Classification System, the American Library Association Interlibrary Loan Code, copyright laws, and local consortia guidelines.

2. The organization develops and enforces data policies, standards, and procedures to define projects and work requirements and to efficiently collect and effectively use data according to the plans. The data are organized and transformed into information in forms useful to decision makers, such as data displayed as graphics, spreadsheets, or tables.

■ Examples of Evidence of Performance—IM.3.1 Through IM.3.3

- Organizationwide policies and procedures
- Departmental policies and procedures
- Data element definitions, abbreviation lists, codes, and data dictionary
- Interviews with staff

■ Scoring for IM.3

This standard is not scored.

■ Scoring for IM.3.1

SCORE 1 Evidence indicates that the organization uses standardized minimum data sets, data definitions, codes, classifications, and terminology.

SCORE 2 Evidence indicates that, with a few, minor exceptions, the organization uses standardized minimum data sets, data definitions, codes, classifications, and terminology.

SCORE 3	Evidence indicates that the organization does not consistently use standardized minimum data sets, data definitions, codes, classifications, and terminology.
SCORE 4	Evidence indicates that the organization seldom uses standardized minimum data sets, data definitions, codes, classifications, and terminology.
SCORE 5	Evidence indicates that the organization does not use standardized minimum data sets, data definitions, codes, classifications, and terminology.

■ Scoring for IM.3.1.1

SCORE 1	Evidence indicates that when organization standards are used, the organization referenced external standards when they were developed.
SCORE 2	Evidence indicates that, with a few minor exceptions, when organization standards are used, the organization referenced external standards when they were developed.
SCORE 3	Evidence indicates that when organization standards are used, the organization did not consistently reference external standards when they were developed.
SCORE 4	Evidence indicates that when organization standards are used, the organization seldom referenced external standards when they were developed.
SCORE 5	Evidence indicates that when organization standards are used, the organization did not reference external standards when they were developed.

■ Scoring for IM.3.2

SCORE 1	The organization collects data in a timely, economical, and efficient manner and with the degree of

accuracy, completeness, and discrimination necessary for their intended use.

SCORE 2 With a few, minor exceptions, the organization collects data in a timely, economical, and efficient manner and with the degree of accuracy, completeness, and discrimination necessary for their intended use.

SCORE 3 The organization does not consistently collect data in a timely, economical, and efficient manner and with the degree of accuracy, completeness, and discrimination necessary for their intended use.

SCORE 4 The organization seldom collects data in a timely, economical, and efficient manner and with the degree of accuracy, completeness, and discrimination necessary for their intended use.

SCORE 5 The organization does not collect data in a timely, economical, and efficient manner and with the degree of accuracy, completeness, and discrimination necessary for their intended use.

▰ Scoring for IM.3.3

SCORE 1 The organization implements mechanisms designed to ascertain that bias in the data is minimized and to assess the data's reliability, validity, and accuracy on an ongoing basis.

SCORE 2 With a few, minor exceptions, the organization implements mechanisms designed to ascertain that bias in the data is minimized and to assess the data's reliability, validity, and accuracy on an ongoing basis.

SCORE 3 The organization does not consistently implement mechanisms designed to ascertain that bias in the data is minimized and to assess the data's reliability, validity, and accuracy on an ongoing basis.

Appendix A   The 1995 *CAMH* Excerpt

SCORE 4   The organization seldom implements mechanisms designed to ascertain that bias in the data is minimized and to assess the data's reliability, validity, and accuracy on an ongoing basis.

SCORE 5   The organization does not implement mechanisms designed to ascertain that bias in the data is minimized and to assess the data's reliability, validity, and accuracy on an ongoing basis.

■ Standards

IM.3.3.1

A 1 2 3 4 5 NA   The organization reviews the completeness, accuracy, and timely completion of information in medical records at least quarterly.

IM.3.3.1.1

A 1 2 3 4 5 NA   The review is performed by, at a minimum, the medical staff in cooperation with nursing, the health information-management (medical record) service, management and administrative services, and representatives of other departments as appropriate.

IM.3.3.1.2

A 1 2 3 4 5 NA   The review determines that each medical record, or a representative sample of records, reflects the diagnosis, diagnostic test results, therapy, the patient's condition and in-hospital progress, and the patient's condition at discharge.

■ Intent of IM.3.3.1 Through IM.3.3.1.2

The review of medical records addresses the presence, accuracy, timeliness, and authentication of the following data and information:

- Identification data;
- Medical history, including the chief complaint; details of the present illness; relevant past, social, and family histories (appropriate to the patient's age); and an inventory by body system;
- A summary of the patient's psychosocial needs, as appropriate to the patient's age;
- A report of relevant physical examinations;
- A statement on the conclusions or impressions drawn from the admission history and physical examination;
- A statement on the course of action planned for the patient for this episode of care and of its periodic review, as appropriate;
- Diagnostic and therapeutic orders;
- Evidence of appropriate informed consent;
- Clinical observations, including the results of therapy;
- Progress notes made by the medical staff and other authorized staff;
- Consultation reports;
- Reports of operative and other invasive procedures, tests, and their results;
- Reports of any diagnostic and therapeutic procedures, such as pathology and clinical laboratory examinations and radiology and nuclear medicine examinations or treatments;
- Records of donation and receipt of transplants and/or implants;
- Final diagnosis(es);
- Conclusions at termination of hospitalization;
- Clinical resumes and discharge summaries;
- Discharge instructions to the patient and/or family; and
- When performed, results of autopsy.

When medical record review is based on a representative sample (that is, a sample representing the practitioners providing care and of the care provided), the review encompasses the organization's or department's full scope of practice, including the most common diagnoses and procedures, and all high-risk procedures. Samples include records of patients currently in the hospital (that is, concurrent review). In addition, medical records from each physician on the medical staff are reviewed at least annually.

It is expected that medical record completion statistics will be available for at least quarterly review and are evident in the reports of this review function, for example, medical record committee minutes or medical executive committee minutes.

■ Scoring for IM.3.3.1

SCORE 1 Medical records are reviewed, as appropriate, for the presence, accuracy, timeliness, and authentication of the data and information listed in the intent.
AND
The review is conducted at least quarterly.

SCORE 2 Medical records are reviewed, as appropriate, for the presence, accuracy, timeliness, and authentication of the data and information listed in the intent.
AND
The review was conducted in three of the four quarters prior to survey.

SCORE 3 Medical records are reviewed, as appropriate, for the presence, accuracy, timeliness, and authentication of the data and information listed in the intent.
AND
The review was conducted in two of the four quarters prior to survey.

SCORE 4 Medical records are reviewed, as appropriate, for the presence, accuracy, timeliness, and authentication of the data and information listed in the intent.
AND
The review was conducted in one of the four quarters prior to survey.

SCORE 5 There is little or no evidence that medical records are reviewed, as appropriate, for the presence, accuracy, timeliness, and authentication of the data and information listed in the intent.

■ Scoring for IM.3.3.1.1

SCORE 1 Evidence indicates that the group reviewing the medical records is composed of the medical staff and other appropriate organization professionals for each quarter in the 12 months prior to survey.

SCORE 2 Evidence indicates that the group reviewing the medical record is composed of the medical staff and other appropriate organization professionals for three out of the four quarters in the 12 months prior to survey.

SCORE 3 Evidence indicates that the group reviewing the medical records is composed of the medical staff and other appropriate organization professionals for two out of the four quarters in the 12 months prior to survey.

SCORE 4 Evidence indicates that the group reviewing the medical records is composed of the medical staff and other appropriate organization professionals for one out of the four quarters in the 12 months prior to survey.
OR
Evidence indicates that medical records are reviewed without medical staff participation.

SCORE 5 There is no evidence that medical records are reviewed.

■ Scoring for IM.3.3.1.2

SCORE 1 Evidence indicates that every medical record, or a sample representing the full scope of services provided, is reviewed.
AND

Reports demonstrate review of the quality of documentation in the medical records, including the diagnosis, results of diagnostic tests, therapy, condition and in-hospital progress, and condition at discharge.

SCORE 2 Evidence indicates that most medical records are reviewed, or the sample of records reviewed is, with a few, minor exceptions, reasonable in size and representative of the type and scope of services provided.

OR

With a few, minor exceptions, reports demonstrate review of the quality of documentation in the medical records, including the diagnosis, results of diagnostic tests, therapy, condition and in-hospital progress, and condition at discharge.

SCORE 3 Evidence indicates that many medical records are not reviewed, or the sample of records reviewed is not representative of the type and scope of services provided.

OR

Reports do not consistently demonstrate review of the quality of documentation in the medical records, including the diagnosis, results of diagnostic tests, therapy, condition and in-hospital progress, and condition at discharge.

SCORE 4 Evidence indicates that few medical records are reviewed, and there is no system for selecting representative samples of medical records.

OR

Reports seldom demonstrate review of the quality of documentation in the medical records, including the diagnosis, results of diagnostic tests, therapy, condition and in-hospital progress, and condition at discharge.

SCORE 5 There is no evidence that medical records are reviewed.
OR
Reports do not demonstrate review of the quality of documentation, including the diagnosis, results of diagnostic tests, therapy, condition and in-hospital progress, and condition at discharge.

■ Standard

IM.4

A 1 2 3 4 5 NA Decision makers and other individuals in the organization who generate, collect, and analyze data and information are educated and trained in the principles of information management.

■ Intent of IM.4

Individuals in the organization who generate, collect, analyze, and use data and information are educated and trained to effectively participate in managing information. This education and training enable these individuals to

- understand security and confidentiality of data and information;
- use measurement instruments, statistical tools, and data analysis methods for transforming data into relevant information;
- collect unbiased data, gathered with a control for confounding or corrected on the basis of acceptable methodologies;
- assist in interpreting data;
- use data and information to help in decision making;
- educate and support the participation of patients and family in care processes; and
- use indicators to assess and improve systems and processes over time.

Individuals are educated and trained as appropriate to their responsibilities, privileges, job descriptions, and data and information needs.

■ Example of Implementation—IM.4

Education in the principles of information management can include how to use tools to transform data into information (for example, flowcharts, histograms, control charts) for decision support and sound sampling methodologies. Knowledge-based information used to support individual or group educational efforts can include literature on statistical and nonstatistical data analysis methods and on the use of information for decision making. Application programs for data analysis and documentation to support their use can be available to those who need them.

■ Examples of Evidence of Performance—IM.4
- Individual performance reports showing continuing education
- Reports and/or minutes documenting data analysis
- Attendance records combined with lecture "outlines"

■ Scoring for IM.4

SCORE 1 Evidence indicates that staff are educated and trained in information management according to their individual needs.

SCORE 2 Evidence indicates that, with a few, minor exceptions, staff are educated and trained in information management according to their individual needs.

SCORE 3 Evidence indicates that staff are not consistently educated and trained in information management according to their individual needs.

SCORE 4 Evidence indicates that staff are seldom educated and trained in information management according to their individual needs.

SCORE 5   Evidence indicates that staff are not educated and trained in information management according to their individual needs.

▪ Standards

IM.5

A 1 2 3 4 5 NA   The transmission of data and information is timely and accurate.

IM.5.1

A 1 2 3 4 5 NA   The format and methods for disseminating data and information are standardized, whenever possible.

▪ Intent of IM.5 and IM.5.1

The transmission of both internally and externally generated data and information to users is accurate and timely, as defined by the need and use for the data and information. The information-management function maintains the integrity of data and information, and provides for communication between the users and suppliers of data and information. The format and methods of disseminating internal data and information are tailored to the organization's and users' needs, and provide for easy retrievability. Data and information exchange formats are standardized whenever possible.

▪ Examples of Implementation—IM.5 Through IM.5.1.1

1. The results of laboratory testing, x-rays, physical therapy treatment, respiratory therapy treatment, and diagnostic testing (for example, Dopplers, Holters, pulmonary function testing) are available to practitioners in a timely manner.
2. Diet orders are timely and are accurately transmitted to the food service department.

3. In the pharmacy, to minimize errors, the use of abbreviations is discouraged, and the use of the leading decimal point is avoided.
4. Telecommunications that provide automated voice messaging as well as electronic transmission of data are used to expedite the role of information.
5. The medical record format is standardized to meet user needs, and the records are accessible 24 hours per day.

■ Examples of Evidence of Performance— IM.5 Through IM.5.1

- Organizationwide policies and procedures
- Departmental policies and procedures
- Interviews with staff
- Approved Code Book

■ Scoring for IM.5

SCORE 1 Evidence indicates that the transmission of data and information is timely and accurate, as defined by need and use.

SCORE 2 Evidence indicates that, with a few, minor exceptions, the transmission of data and information is timely and accurate, as defined by need and use.

SCORE 3 Evidence indicates that the transmission of data and information is not consistently timely and accurate, as defined by need and use.

SCORE 4 Evidence indicates that the transmission of data and information is seldom timely and accurate, as defined by need and use.

SCORE 5 Evidence indicates that the transmission of data and information is not timely and accurate, as defined by need and use.

■ Scoring for IM.5.1

SCORE 1   The format and methods for disseminating data and information meet users' needs and are standardized, whenever possible, to facilitate interpretation.

SCORE 2   With a few, minor exceptions, the format and methods for disseminating data and information meet users' needs and are standardized, whenever possible, to facilitate interpretation.

SCORE 3   The format and methods for disseminating data and information do not consistently meet users' needs and are not consistently standardized, whenever possible, to facilitate interpretation.

SCORE 4   The format and methods for disseminating data and information seldom meet users' needs and are not standardized to facilitate interpretation.

SCORE 5   The format and methods for disseminating data and information do not meet users' needs and are not standardized to facilitate interpretation.

■ Standards

IM.6

A 1 2 3 4 5 NA   The information-management function enables the combination of data and information; makes information from one system (clinical and/or organizational) available to another; provides reports; clarifies and interprets data and information; and enables linkage of patient care and nonpatient care data and information over time among the organization's departments and provider resources for all care settings.

IM.6.1

A 1 2 3 4 5 NA   The retention time of medical record information is determined by law and regulation and by its use for patient care, legal, research, and/or educational purposes.

IM.6.2

A 1 2 3 4 5 NA There are internal linkages among information-management processes related to the important patient care and organizational functions described in this Manual.

IM.6.3

A 1 2 3 4 5 NA The organization has access to external databases* and bodies of expert health-related, administrative, and research knowledge, as required by its information-management needs.

■ Intent of IM.6 Through IM.6.3

The information-management process gathers information from various sources; accesses and provides longitudinal data and information; uses internal and external linkages, as needed; analyzes situations based on this information; and makes decisions based on this analysis. Systems for accessing external information are linked to systems of internal information as appropriate. The information-management system provides for the interface of patient care data and clinical literature, and organizational data and management literature. The retention of data and information depends on the need to support patient care, organizational management, legal records, research, and education and the need to conform to applicable law and regulation.

■ Examples of Implementation—IM.6 Through IM.6.3

1. The ability to link clinical and financial information is a valuable way to assess resource use in the health care delivery process. Other examples could be long-term knowledge of staffing, patient volume, length of stay, and payment records.

---

* **database** A collection of stored data.

The collection of organizationally determined performance indicators (including adverse events) can be used to assess and improve clinical, managerial, and support processes.

Examples of internal information systems that have potential for linkage include clinical information systems (for example, medical record, pharmacy, laboratory systems); the systems for managing knowledge-based information (for example, professional library system); information systems for tracking, aggregating, and comparing internal information; administrative and financial information systems; instructional systems (for example, patient and family, staff); research information systems; and communication and office support systems (for example, word processing, electronic mail).

2. In computerized organizations, Health Level 7 (HL7) standards are used for within-institution transmission of orders, clinical observations and clinical data (including test results), admission transfer and discharge records, and charge and billing information. For example, HL7 facilitates the transfer of laboratory results, pharmacy data, and other information for a patient to a central hospital system without concern for whether such systems are supplied by the same vendor or manufacturer.

■ Examples of Evidence of Performance— IM.6 Through IM.6.3

- Organizationwide policies and procedures
- Departmental policies and procedures
- Interviews with staff involved in collecting, analyzing, and using data and information throughout the organization
- Agreements with reference database(s) and other external data and information resources for access and/or participation

■ Scoring for IM.6

SCORE 1   Evidence indicates that for both patient care and nonpatient care services, the organization's information-management function can

- coordinate collection of information;
- make information from one system available to another;
- organize data;
- analyze data;
- interpret and clarify the data and information; and
- access and provide longitudinal data and information.

SCORE 2 Evidence indicates that for patient care services, the organization's information-management function can perform the items listed in Score 1; however, for nonpatient care services, the organization's information-management function cannot consistently perform the items listed in Score 1.

SCORE 3 Evidence indicates that for patient care services, the organization's information-management function cannot consistently perform the items listed in Score 1.
OR
Evidence indicates that for nonpatient care services, the organization's information-management function can seldom perform the items listed in Score 1.

SCORE 4 Evidence indicates that for patient care services, the organization's information-management function can seldom perform the items listed in Score 1.
AND
Evidence indicates that for nonpatient care services, the organization's information-management function cannot perform the items listed in Score 1.

SCORE 5 Evidence indicates that for both patient care and nonpatient care services, the organization's information-management function cannot perform the items listed in Score 1.

■ Scoring for IM.6.1

SCORE 1 The organization follows its policy on medical record information retention.
AND
The policy addresses the length of time information is retained, which is determined by the following five factors:
- Law and regulation;
- Its use for patient care;
- Its use for legal purposes;
- Its use for research; and
- Its use for education.

SCORE 2 With a few, minor exceptions, the organization follows its policy on medical record information retention.
OR
The policy addresses the length of time information is retained, but it considers only four of the five factors listed in Score 1.

SCORE 3 The organization does not consistently follow its policy on medical record information retention.
OR
The policy addresses the length of time information is retained, but it considers only three of the five factors listed in Score 1.

SCORE 4 The organization seldom follows its policy on medical record information retention.
OR
The policy addresses the length of time information is retained, but it considers only one or two of the five factors listed in Score 1.

SCORE 5 The organization does not follow its policy on medical record information retention.
OR

The policy does not address the five factors listed in Score 1.

■ Scoring for IM.6.2

SCORE 1 Evidence indicates that there are internal linkages of data and information processes *within* and *between* the patient care and the organizational functions described in the *CAMH*.

SCORE 2 Evidence indicates that there are internal linkages of data and information processes *within* the patient care and the organizational functions described in the *CAMH*, but there is inconsistent linkage *between* these functions.

SCORE 3 Evidence indicates that there are inconsistent internal linkages of data and information processes *within* the patient care and the organizational functions described in the *CAMH*, but there is minimal linkage *between* these functions.

SCORE 4 Evidence indicates that there are minimal internal linkages of data and information processes *within* the patient care and the organizational functions described in the *CAMH*, and there is no linkage *between* these functions.

SCORE 5 Evidence indicates that there are no internal linkages of data and information processes *within* and *between* the patient care and the organizational functions described in the *CAMH*.

■ Scoring for IM.6.3

SCORE 1 The organization has access to external databases and bodies of knowledge-based resources as required by its information-management needs.

SCORE 2 With a few, minor exceptions, the organization has access to external databases and bodies of knowledge-based resources as required by its information-management needs.

SCORE 3 The organization does not have consistent access to external databases and bodies of knowledge-based resources as required by its information-management needs.

SCORE 4 The organization seldom has access to external databases and bodies of knowledge-based resources as required by its information-management needs.

SCORE 5 The organization does not have access to external databases and bodies of knowledge-based resources as required by its information-management needs.

EXHIBIT 5 Aggregation Summary

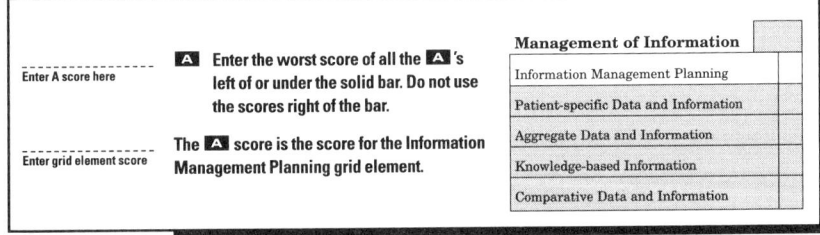

Patient-Specific Data and Information

Standards

IM.7 *The information-management function provides for the definition, capture, analysis, transformation, transmission, and reporting of individual patient-specific data and information related to the process(es) and/or of the outcome(s) of the patient's care.*

IM.7.1
A 1 2 3 4 5 NA The organization initiates and maintains a medical record* for every individual assessed or treated. The medical record incorporates information from subsequent contacts between the patient and the organization.

IM.7.1.1
A 1 2 3 4 5 NA Entries in medical records are made only by individuals authorized to do so as specified in organization and medical staff policies.

IM.7.2 *The medical record contains sufficient information to identify the patient, support the diagnosis, justify the treatment, document the course and results accurately, and facilitate continuity of care among health care providers. Each medical record contains at least the following:*

IM.7.2.1
A 1 2 3 4 5 NA The patient's name, address, date of birth, and the name of any legally authorized representative;

IM.7.2.2
A 1 2 3 4 5 NA The patient's legal status, for patients receiving mental health services;

IM.7.2.3
A 1 2 3 4 5 NA Emergency care provided to the patient prior to arrival, if any;

IM.7.2.4 *The record and findings of the patient's assessment (see the "Assessment of Patients" chapter in the* CAMH*);*

IM.7.2.5
B 1 2 3 4 5 NA A statement of the conclusions or impressions drawn from the medical history and physical examination;

---

* **medical record** The account compiled by physicians and other health care professionals of a variety of patient health information, such as the patient's assessment findings, treatment details, and progress notes.

IM.7.2.6
B 1 2 3 4 5 NA   The diagnosis or diagnostic impression;

IM.7.2.7
B 1 2 3 4 5 NA   The reason(s) for admission or treatment;

IM.7.2.8 *The goals of treatment and the treatment plan;*

IM.7.2.9
A 1 2 3 4 5 NA   Evidence of known advance directives;

IM.7.2.10
A 1 2 3 4 5 NA   Evidence of informed consent for procedures and treatments for which informed consent is required by organizational policy;

IM.7.2.11
A 1 2 3 4 5 NA   Diagnostic and therapeutic orders, if any;

IM.7.2.12
A 1 2 3 4 5 NA   All diagnostic and therapeutic procedures and tests performed and the results;

IM.7.2.13 *All operative and other invasive procedures performed, using acceptable disease and operative terminology that includes etiology, as appropriate;*

IM.7.2.14
A 1 2 3 4 5 NA   Progress notes made by the medical staff and other authorized individuals;

IM.7.2.15
C 1 2 3 4 5 NA   All reassessments, when necessary;

IM.7.2.16
C 1 2 3 4 5 NA   Clinical observations;

IM.7.2.17
C 1 2 3 4 5 NA   The response to the care provided;

IM.7.2.18
A 1 2 3 4 5 NA   Consultation reports;

IM.7.2.19
A 1 2 3 4 5 NA   Every medication ordered or prescribed for an inpatient;

IM.7.2.20
A 1 2 3 4 5 NA   Every dose of medication administered and any adverse drug reaction;

IM.7.2.21
A 1 2 3 4 5 NA   Every medication dispensed to or prescribed for an ambulatory patient or an inpatient on discharge;

IM.7.2.22
A 1 2 3 4 5 NA   All relevant diagnoses established during the course of care; and

IM.7.2.23
A 1 2 3 4 5 NA   Any referrals and communications made to external or internal care providers and to community agencies.

■ Intent of IM.7 Through IM.7.2.23

The information-management function provides for the use of patient-specific data and information to
- facilitate patient care;
- serve as a financial and legal record;
- help in clinical research; and
- support decision analysis.

Patient-specific data and information also provide a basis for professional and organizational performance improvement. A heterogeneous group—administrative staff, ancillary departments, and direct care providers—provides and uses this information. The system recalls historical data about a specific patient as well as accesses data about current encounters. To facilitate consistency and continuity in patient care, very specific data and information are required, as outlined in the standards.

The environment in which patient-specific information is provided supports timely, accurate, secure, and confidential recording and use of patient-specific information.

Examples of Implementation—IM.7 Through IM.7.2.23.1

1. Nursing care data related to patient assessments, nursing diagnoses and/or patient needs, nursing interventions, and patient outcomes are permanently integrated into the medical record.
2. The record of a patient receiving radiation oncology therapy reflects a histologically substantiated diagnosis. The patient's medical record includes interpretations of radiology studies and descriptions of invasive procedures.
3. Respiratory care services are provided to patients in accordance with a written prescription by the physician responsible for the patient and are documented in the patient's medical record.
4. The medical record documents progress toward rehabilitation goal achievement and includes the results of the planned therapeutic intervention and the patient's responses to such interventions.
5. Procedures, such as the use of perioperative blood-saving techniques including hemodilution, intraoperative collection and reinfusion, and postoperative drainage and reinfusion, are documented thoroughly in the patient's medical record so that adverse consequences can be properly assessed.

6. The patient's medical record documents diagnostic and therapeutic orders, including diet orders, and clinical observations, including height and weight. These parameters are essential for conducting patient nutrition assessments, drug dosing, and certain diagnostic tests.
7. The patient's response to the care provided is documented in the medical record. For example, staff need to assess and document the patient's response to antibiotics or pain medication. Also, when specific care goals are developed as part of the initial assessment process, progress or lack of progress towards goal achievement is documented.
8. Written organizational policies and procedures address the use of standing orders. For instance, in an intensive care unit (ICU), the medical director of the unit has approved a set of standing orders to be implemented when qualified ICU registered nurses identify warning dysrhythmias.

■ Examples of Evidence of Performance— IM.7 Through IM.7.2.23

- Organizationwide policies and procedures
- Departmental policies and procedures
- Medical staff rules and regulations
- Review of medical records from all care sites and all clinical services provided by the organization, including records of discharged patients and patients currently in the hospital or receiving ambulatory services

■ Scoring for IM.7
This standard is not scored.

■ Scoring for IM.7.1

SCORE 1 The organization maintains a medical record for all patients its treats in any setting.

SCORE 5 The organization does not maintain a medical record for one or more patients it treats.

■ Scoring for IM.7.1.1

SCORE 1 The organization has established policies that define who is allowed to make entries in the medical record, and these policies are followed.

SCORE 3 The organization has established policies that define who is allowed to make entries in the medical record, but these policies are inconsistently followed.

SCORE 5 The organization has not established policies that define who is allowed to make entries in the medical record.
OR
If the organization has established policies, they are not followed.

■ Scoring for IM.7.2

This standard is not scored.

■ Scoring for IM.7.2.1 Through IM.7.2.23

Note: IM.7.2.4 is scored in the "Assessment of Patients" chapter in the CAMH; IM.7.2.8 is scored at TX.1; and IM.7.2.13 is scored at IM.7.4.2. The following set of scoring guidelines applies to each of the remaining standards in this set.

SCORE 1 91% to 100% of medical records reviewed contain the stated requirements.

SCORE 2 76% to 90% of medical records reviewed contain the stated requirements.

SCORE 3 51% to 75% of medical records reviewed contain the stated requirements.

SCORE 4 26% to 50% of medical records reviewed contain the stated requirements.

SCORE 5 Fewer than 26% of medical records reviewed contain the stated requirements.

▪ Standards

IM.7.3

A 1 2 3 4 5 NA   At discharge from inpatient care, a clinical resume concisely summarizes the reason for hospitalization, the significant findings, the procedures performed and treatment rendered, the patient's condition on discharge, and any specific instructions given to the patient and/or family, as pertinent.

IM.7.3.1

A 1 2 3 4 5 NA   A final progress note is substituted for the resume only for those patients with problems and interventions of a minor nature (as defined by the medical staff) who require less than a 48-hour period of hospitalization and in the case of normal newborn infants and uncomplicated obstetric deliveries.

IM.7.3.2

A 1 2 3 4 5 NA   A transfer summary may be substituted for the resume if the patient is transferred to a different level of hospitalization or residential care within the organization.

▪ Intent of IM.7.3 Through IM.7.3.2

To provide important information concisely to the medical record's other users and facilitate continuity of care, a clinical resume is included in the record at discharge (or in the circumstances outlined in IM.7.3.1, a final progress note). When a patient is transferred from one level of care (for example, hospital) to another level of care (for example, residential or partial hospitalization) within the same organization, and the caregivers change, a transfer summary may be substituted for the clinical resume. When the caregivers remain the same, a progress note may be sufficient. When the patient is discharged to ambulatory (outpatient) care, the medical record includes a clinical resume of the previous levels of care.

■ Scoring for IM.7.3

SCORE 1 91% to 100% of medical records reviewed contain a discharge summary that includes the following factors:
- The reason for hospitalization;
- The significant findings;
- The procedures performed and treatment rendered;
- The patient's condition on discharge; and
- Any specific instructions given to the patient and/or family, as pertinent.

SCORE 2 76% to 90% of medical records reviewed contain the factors listed in Score 1.

SCORE 3 51% to 75% of medical records reviewed contain the factors listed in Score 1.

SCORE 4 26% to 50% of medical records reviewed contain the factors listed in Score 1.

SCORE 5 Fewer than 26% of medical records reviewed contain the factors listed in Score 1.

■ Scoring for IM.7.3.1

SCORE 1 Final progress notes, when substituted for the clinical resume, consistently meet the requirements stated in the standard.

SCORE 3 Final progress notes, when substituted for the clinical resume, inconsistently meet the requirements stated in the standard.

SCORE 5 Final progress notes, when substituted for the clinical resume, do not meet any of the requirements stated in the standard.

■ Scoring for IM.7.3.2

SCORE 1 Transfer summaries, when used, consistently meet the requirements stated in the standard and the intent.

SCORE 3 Transfer summaries, when used, inconsistently meet the requirements stated in the standard and the intent.

SCORE 5 Transfer summaries, when used, do not meet any of the requirements stated in the standard and the intent.

■ Standards

IM.7.4 *The medical record of patients undergoing operative or other invasive procedures and/or anesthesia includes the additional following information:*

IM.7.4.1

A 1 2 3 4 5 NA The licensed independent practitioner who is responsible for the patient records a preoperative diagnosis prior to surgery.

IM.7.4.2

A 1 2 3 4 5 NA Operative reports are dictated or written in the medical record immediately after surgery and describe the findings, the technical procedures used, the specimen(s) removed, the postoperative diagnosis, and the name of the primary surgeon and any assistants.

IM.7.4.2.1

A 1 2 3 4 5 NA The completed operative report is authenticated* by the surgeon and filed in the medical record as soon as possible after surgery.

---

* **authenticate** To prove authorship, for example, by written signature, identifiable initials, or a computer key.

IM.7.4.2.2

A 1 2 3 4 5 NA When the operative report is not placed in the medical record immediately after surgery (for example, there is a transcription and/or filing delay), an operative progress note is entered in the medical record immediately after surgery to provide pertinent information for any individual required to attend to the patient.

IM.7.4.3 *Postoperative documentation includes at least a record of*

IM.7.4.3.1 *vital signs and level of consciousness;*

IM.7.4.3.2 *medications (including intravenous fluids) and blood and blood components;*

IM.7.4.3.3 *any unusual events or postoperative complications, including blood transfusion reactions, and the management of those events;*

IM.7.4.3.4

A 1 2 3 4 5 NA identification of who provided direct patient care nursing services and who supervised that care if it was provided by someone other than a qualified registered nurse;

IM.7.4.3.5 *the patient's discharge from the postanesthesia care area by the responsible licensed independent practitioner or by the use of relevant discharge criteria; and*

IM.7.4.3.5.1

A 1 2 3 4 5 NA The criteria are approved by the medical staff and rigorously applied to determine the patient's readiness for discharge.

IM.7.4.3.6

A 1 2 3 4 5 NA the name of the licensed independent practitioner responsible for the discharge.

■ Intent of IM.7.4 Through IM.7.4.3.6

In addition to the specific information required in all medical records (IM.7 through IM.7.3.2), a record is kept of all aspects of a surgical patient's preoperative, operative, and postoperative events. The record includes the preoperative diagnosis, a complete description of the surgical procedure and findings, the identity of all practitioners involved in the process, the postoperative course, evidence of the patient's readiness for discharge from the postanesthesia care area, and the discharge. Operative reports are thoroughly and consistently recorded in the medical record in accordance with organizational policies and procedures and applicable state laws. This requirement applies to the medical records of all outpatients and inpatients, including donors and recipients of organs and tissues.

■ Scoring for IM.7.4

This standard is not scored.

■ Scoring for IM.7.4.1

SCORE 1 100% of medical records reviewed of patients who have undergone operative or other invasive procedures and/or have received anesthesia services, including donors and recipients of organs and tissues, contain a preoperative diagnosis by a licensed independent practitioner.

SCORE 2 95% to 99% of medical records reviewed of patients who have undergone operative or other invasive procedures and/or have received anesthesia services, including donors and recipients of organs and tissues, contain a preoperative diagnosis by a licensed independent practitioner.

SCORE 3 90% to 94% of medical records reviewed of patients who have undergone operative or other invasive procedures and/or have received anesthesia services, including donors and recipients of organs and tissues, contain a preoperative diagnosis by a licensed independent practitioner.

SCORE 4 80% to 89% of medical records reviewed of patients who have undergone operative or other invasive procedures and/or have received anesthesia services, including donors and recipients of organs and tissues, contain a preoperative diagnosis by a licensed independent practitioner.

SCORE 5 Fewer than 80% of medical records reviewed of patients who have undergone operative or other invasive procedures and/or have received anesthesia services, including donors and recipients of organs and tissues, contain a preoperative diagnosis by a licensed independent practitioner.

■ Scoring for IM.7.4.2

SCORE 1 100% of medical records reviewed of patients who have undergone operative or other invasive procedures and/or have received anesthesia services, including donors and recipients of organs and tissues, contain an operative report recorded in accordance with organizational policies and procedures and applicable state laws.
AND
All five of the requirements listed in the standard appear in the operative report.

SCORE 2 90% to 99% of medical records reviewed of patients who have undergone operative or other invasive procedures and/or have received anesthesia services, including donors and recipients of organs and tissues, contain an operative report recorded in accordance with organizational policies and procedures and applicable state laws.
OR

Four of the five requirements listed in the standard appear in the operative report.

SCORE 3 76% to 89% of medical records reviewed of patients who have undergone operative or other invasive procedures and/or have received anesthesia services, including donors and recipients of organs and tissues, contain an operative report recorded in accordance with organizational policies and procedures and applicable state laws.

OR

Three of the five requirements listed in the standard appear in the operative report.

SCORE 4 51% to 75% of medical records reviewed of patients who have undergone operative or other invasive procedures and/or have received anesthesia services, including donors and recipients of organs and tissues, contain an operative report recorded in accordance with organizational policies and procedures and applicable state laws.

OR

Two of the five requirements listed in the standard appear in the operative report.

SCORE 5 Fewer than 51% of medical records reviewed of patients who have undergone operative or other invasive procedures and/or have received anesthesia services, including donors and recipients of organs and tissues, contain an operative report recorded in accordance with organizational policies and procedures and applicable state laws.

OR

One or none of the five requirements listed in the standard appears in the operative report.

■ Scoring for IM.7.4.2.1

SCORE 1 100% of medical records reviewed of patients who have undergone operative or other invasive procedures and/or have received anesthesia services, including donors and recipients of organs and tissues, contain a completed operative report authenticated and dated by the surgeon.

SCORE 2 90% to 99% of medical records reviewed of patients who have undergone operative or other invasive procedures and/or have received anesthesia services, including donors and recipients of organs and tissues, contain a completed operative report authenticated and dated by the surgeon.

SCORE 3 76% to 89% of medical records reviewed of patients who have undergone operative or other invasive procedures and/or have received anesthesia services, including donors and recipients of organs and tissues, contain a completed operative report authenticated and dated by the surgeon.

SCORE 4 51% to 75% of medical records reviewed of patients who have undergone operative or other invasive procedures and/or have received anesthesia services, including donors and recipients of organs and tissues, contain a completed operative report authenticated and dated by the surgeon.

SCORE 5 Fewer than 51% of medical records reviewed of patients who have undergone operative or other invasive procedures and/or have received anesthesia services, including donors and recipients of organs and tissues, contain a completed operative report authenticated and dated by the surgeon.

Scoring for IM.7.4.2.2

SCORE 1 100% of medical records reviewed of patients who have undergone operative or other invasive procedures and/or have received anesthesia services, including donors and recipients of organs and tissues, indicate that the completed operative reports were dictated or written immediately after surgery. In cases in which evidence shows that a transcription or filing delay made it impossible to produce an operative report within six hours following surgery, an operative progress note was filed in the medical record containing pertinent information needed by any individual who might attend the patient.

SCORE 2 90% to 99% of medical records reviewed of patients who have undergone operative or other invasive procedures and/or have received anesthesia services, including donors and recipients of organs and tissues, indicate that the completed operative reports were dictated or written immediately after surgery. In cases in which evidence shows that a transcription or filing delay made it impossible to produce an operative report within six hours following surgery, an operative progress note was filed in the medical record containing pertinent information needed by any individual who might attend the patient.

SCORE 3 76% to 89% of medical records reviewed of patients who have undergone operative or other invasive procedures and/or have received anesthesia services, including donors and recipients of organs and tissues, indicate that the completed operative reports were dictated or written immediately after surgery. In cases in which evidence shows that a transcription or filing delay made it impossible to produce an operative report within six hours following surgery, an operative progress note was filed in the medical record containing pertinent information needed by any individual who might attend the patient.

SCORE 4 51% to 75% of medical records reviewed of patients who have undergone operative or other invasive procedures and/or have received anesthesia services, including donors and recipients of organs and tissues, indicate that the completed operative reports were dictated or written immediately after surgery. In cases in which evidence shows that a transcription or filing delay made it impossible to produce an operative report within six hours following surgery, an operative progress note was filed in the medical record containing pertinent information needed by any individual who might attend the patient.

SCORE 5 Fewer than 51% of medical records reviewed of patients who have undergone operative or other invasive procedures and/or have received anesthesia services, including donors and recipients of organs and tissues, indicate that the completed operative reports were dictated or written immediately after surgery. In cases in which evidence shows that a transcription or filing delay made it impossible to produce an operative report within six hours following surgery, an operative progress note was filed in the medical record containing pertinent information needed by any individual who might attend the patient.

■ Scoring for IM.7.4.3

This standard is not scored.

■ Scoring for IM.7.4.3.1 Through IM.7.4.3.3

These standards are scored in the "Care of Patients" chapter of the *CAMH*.

■ Scoring for IM.7.4.3.4 and IM.7.4.3.6

Note: *The following set of guidelines applies to each standard IM.7.4.3.4 and IM.7.4.3.6.*

SCORE 1 91% to 100% of medical records reviewed of patients who have undergone operative or other invasive procedures and/or have received anesthesia services, including donors and recipients of organs and tissue, contain the stated requirements.

SCORE 2 76% to 90% of medical records reviewed of patients who have undergone operative or other invasive procedures and/or have received anesthesia services, including donors and recipients of organs and tissue, contain the stated requirements.

SCORE 3 51% to 75% of medical records reviewed of patients who have undergone operative or other invasive procedures and/or have received anesthesia services, including donors and recipients of organs and tissue, contain the stated requirements.

SCORE 4 26% to 50% of medical records reviewed of patients who have undergone operative or other invasive procedures and/or have received anesthesia services, including donors and recipients of organs and tissue, contain the stated requirements.

SCORE 5 Fewer than 26% of medical records reviewed of patients who have undergone operative or other invasive procedures and/or have received anesthesia services, including donors and recipients of organs and tissue, contain the stated requirements.

Scoring for IM.7.4.3.5
This standard is scored at TX.2.4.1.

Scoring for IM.7.4.3.5.1

SCORE 1 Relevant discharge criteria are approved by the medical staff.
AND
The criteria are rigorously applied to determine the patient's readiness for discharge.

SCORE 5 Relevant discharge criteria are not approved by the medical staff.
OR
The criteria are not rigorously applied to determine the patient's readiness for discharge.

Standards

IM.7.5

A 1 2 3 4 5 NA The medical record for patients receiving continuing ambulatory care services includes a list of known significant diagnoses, conditions, procedures, drug allergies, and medications.

IM.7.5.1

A 1 2 3 4 5 NA The list is initiated and maintained for each patient by the third visit.

Intent of IM.7.5 and IM.7.5.1

To promote continuity of care among providers or over time for a single provider, a record for patients receiving ambulatory care services is maintained and provides easy access to significant information. The specific requirement for a list (often referred to as a "summary list") is applicable only to patients who are seen for continuing ambulatory care, that is, three or more visits. The

information is in the same location in all records to help the practitioner(s) quickly find the information. The list contains
- known significant medical diagnoses and conditions;
- known significant operative and invasive procedures;
- known adverse and allergic drug reactions; and
- medications known to be prescribed for and/or used by the patient.

Known refers to information gathered as part of the ambulatory care assessment and treatment. If a patient is seen in more than one clinic in the organization and if each clinic maintains a separate medical record, the list in each record indicates, at a minimum, that there is information in another record.

■ Scoring for IM.7.5

SCORE 1 A list containing at least the four items listed in the intent, as applicable, is in 91% to 100% of medical records reviewed of ambulatory care patients.

SCORE 2 A list containing at least the four items listed in the intent, as applicable, is in 76% to 90% of medical records reviewed of ambulatory care patients.

SCORE 3 A list containing at least the four items listed in the intent, as applicable, is in 51% to 75% of medical records reviewed of ambulatory care patients.

SCORE 4 A list containing at least the four items listed in the intent, as applicable, is in 26% to 50% of medical records reviewed of ambulatory care patients.

SCORE 5 A list containing at least the four items listed in the intent, as applicable, is in fewer than 26% of medical records reviewed of ambulatory care patients.

■ Scoring for IM.7.5.1

SCORE 1 A list containing at least the four items listed in the intent, as applicable, is in 91% to 100% of medical records reviewed of ambulatory care patients who have been seen in the ambulatory care service on at least three occasions.

SCORE 2   A list containing at least the four items listed in the intent, as applicable, is in 76% to 90% of medical records reviewed of ambulatory care patients who have been seen in the ambulatory care service on at least three occasions.

SCORE 3   A list containing at least the four items listed in the intent, as applicable, is in 51% to 75% of medical records reviewed of ambulatory care patients who have been seen in the ambulatory care service on at least three occasions.

SCORE 4   A list containing at least the four items listed in the intent, as applicable, is in 26% to 50% of medical records reviewed of ambulatory care patients who have been seen in the ambulatory care service on at least three occasions.

SCORE 5   A list containing at least the four items listed in the intent, as applicable, is in fewer than 26% of medical records reviewed of ambulatory care patients who have been seen in the ambulatory care service on at least three occasions.

■ Standards

IM.7.6 *When emergency care is provided,*

IM.7.6.1 *the following additional information is required in the medical record:*

IM.7.6.1.1
A 1 2 3 4 5 NA   Time and means of arrival;

IM.7.6.1.2

A 1 2 3 4 5 NA The patient's leaving against medical advice; and

IM.7.6.1.3

A 1 2 3 4 5 NA Conclusions at termination of treatment, including final disposition, condition at discharge, and any instructions for follow-up care.

IM.7.6.2

A 1 2 3 4 5 NA When authorized by the patient or his or her legally authorized representative, a copy of the record of emergency services provided is available to the practitioner or medical organization responsible for follow-up care.

■ Intent of IM.7.6 Through IM.7.6.2

In addition to those items that all medical records are required to contain (IM.7.1 through IM.7.3.2), the medical records of patients who have received emergency care contain additional information related to the emergency visit.

■ Scoring for IM.7.6 and IM.7.6.1

These standards are not scored.

■ Scoring for IM.7.6.1.1

SCORE 1 91% to 100% of medical records reviewed contain the time and means of arrival.

SCORE 2 76% to 90% of medical records reviewed contain the time and means of arrival.

SCORE 3 51% to 75% of medical records reviewed contain the time and means of arrival.

SCORE 4 26% to 50% of medical records reviewed contain the time and means of arrival.

SCORE 5 Fewer than 26% of medical records reviewed contain the time and means of arrival.

■ Scoring for IM.7.6.1.2

SCORE 1 91% to 100% of medical records reviewed record the patient's leaving against medical advice, when appropriate.

SCORE 2 76% to 90% of medical records reviewed record the patient's leaving against medical advice, when appropriate.

SCORE 3 51% to 75% of medical records reviewed record the patient's leaving against medical advice, when appropriate.

SCORE 4 26% to 50% of medical records reviewed record the patient's leaving against medical advice, when appropriate.

SCORE 5 Fewer than 26% of medical records reviewed record the patient's leaving against medical advice, when appropriate.

■ Scoring for IM.7.6.1.3

SCORE 1 91% to 100% of medical records reviewed contain conclusions at termination of treatment, including final disposition, condition at discharge, and any instructions for follow-up care.

SCORE 2 76% to 90% of medical records reviewed contain conclusions at termination of treatment, including final disposition, condition at discharge, and any instructions for follow-up care.

SCORE 3 51% to 75% of medical records reviewed contain conclusions at termination of treatment, including

Appendix A The 1995 *CAMH* Excerpt

final disposition, condition at discharge, and any instructions for follow-up care.

SCORE 4 26% to 50% of medical records reviewed contain conclusions at termination of treatment, including final disposition, condition at discharge, and instructions for follow-up care.

SCORE 5 Fewer than 26% of medical records reviewed contain conclusions at termination of treatment, including final disposition, condition at discharge, and any instructions for follow-up care.

Scoring for IM.7.6.2

SCORE 1 The organization consistently uses a mechanism designed to make a copy of the record of emergency services available to the practitioner or organization responsible for follow-up care when authorized by the patient or the legally authorized representative.

SCORE 3 The organization has a mechanism in place, but does not consistently use it, to make a copy of the record of emergency services available to the practitioner or organization responsible for follow-up care when authorized by the patient or the legally authorized representative.

SCORE 5 The organization does not have a mechanism in place and does not make a copy of the record of emergency services available to the practitioner or organization responsible for follow-up care when authorized by the patient or the legally authorized representative.

Standards

IM.7.7 *Medical record data and information are managed in a timely manner.*

IM.7.7.1

A 1 2 3 4 5 NA   All significant clinical information pertaining to a patient is entered into the medical record as soon as possible after its occurrence.

IM.7.7.2

A 1 2 3 4 5 NA   Medical records of discharged patients must be completed within a time period specified in medical staff rules and regulations, not to exceed 30 days.

■ Intent of IM.7.7 Through IM.7.7.2

The medical record needs timely entries if it is to be valuable in the patient's concurrent care. Documentation in the medical record of the history, physical examination, and operative reports is particularly important. At discharge, a complete medical record is important; however, the time frame is less critical. The medical record is complete when (1) its contents reflect the diagnosis, diagnostic test results, therapy, patient's condition and in-hospital progress, and condition at discharge; and (2) its contents, including any required clinical resume or final progress notes, are assembled and authenticated, and all final diagnoses and complications are recorded without the use of symbols or abbreviations.

Note: *A medical record is defined as "delinquent" when it has not been completed within a specific time period following patient discharge. This time period is specified in the medical staff's rules and regulations and cannot exceed 30 days. Hospital staff should complete medical records as soon as possible after discharge so that information can promptly be retrieved for clinical, legal, or performance improvement purposes.*

■ Examples of Implementation— IM.7.7 Through IM.7.7.2

1. All inpatient records reflect that a medical history and physical examination are completed on each patient within 24 hours of admission (see the "Assessment of Patients" chapter of the *CAMH*). This time frame applies for weekend, holiday, and

weekday admissions. A durable, legible original or reproduction of a medical history and a completed physical assessment, obtained in the office of a physician or an oral and maxillofacial surgeon on the medical staff, completed or thoroughly updated within 30 days before admission, is acceptable provided that the patient's condition did not significantly change during the period between documentation of the history and physical examination and admission to the hospital. When significant changes have occurred, they are recorded at the time of admission. If a patient is readmitted for treatment of the same or a related problem within 30 days following discharge from the hospital, an interval history and physical examination report reflecting any subsequent changes may be used in the medical record, provided that the original information is included in the record.
2. Treatment plans (records) are updated when the patient's needs and response to treatment change.
3. Treatment plans (records) are updated when blood transfusions are provided at home or in an ambulatory care setting (or outside a hospital) and when any transfusion reactions are observed.
4. When an autopsy is performed, provisional anatomic diagnoses are recorded in the medical record within three days, and the complete protocol is included in the record within 60 days, unless the medical staff establishes exceptions for special studies.

■ Examples of Evidence of Performance— IM.7.7 Through IM.7.7.2

- Departmental policies and procedures
- Medical staff rules and regulations
- Review of medical records from all care sites and all clinical services provided by the organization, including records of discharged patients and patients currently in the hospital or receiving ambulatory services

- Data relating to timeliness of completion of medical records for at least the year prior to survey
- Reports of the medical record review function (IM.3.3.1)

■ Scoring for IM.7.7
This standard is not scored.

■ Scoring for IM.7.7.1

SCORE 1   91% to 100% of medical records reviewed indicate that significant clinical information is entered within the appropriate time frames.
AND
The organization has a policy or mechanism designed to ensure timely entries.

SCORE 2   76% to 90% of medical records reviewed indicate that significant clinical information is entered within the appropriate time frames.
AND
The organization has a policy or mechanism designed to ensure timely entries.

SCORE 3   51% to 75% of medical records reviewed indicate that significant clinical information is entered within the appropriate time frames.
OR
The organization does not have a policy or mechanism designed to ensure timely entries.

SCORE 4   26% to 50% of medical records reviewed indicate that significant clinical information is entered within the appropriate time frames.

SCORE 5   Fewer than 26% of medical records reviewed indicate that significant clinical information is entered within the appropriate time frames.

■ Scoring for IM.7.7.2

SCORE 1 The average number of delinquent records, based on at least four (quarterly) determinations, is less than 50% of the average monthly discharges (AMD), and no single determination exceeds 50% of the AMD.

AND

The average number of medical records that are delinquent due to the absence of a medical history and physical examination, based on at least four (quarterly) determinations, is fewer than nine, or 2% of the AMD (whichever is greater).

AND

The average number of medical records delinquent due to the absence of an operative report, based on at least four (quarterly) determinations is fewer than nine, or 2% of the average monthly operative procedures (AMOP) (whichever is greater).

SCORE 2 The average number of delinquent records, based on at least four (quarterly) determinations, is fewer than 50% of the AMD, but one or more of the quarterly determinations exceeds 50% of the AMD, but none exceeds 100%.

OR

The average number of medical records that are delinquent due to the absence of a medical history and physical examination, based on at least four (quarterly) determinations, is fewer than nine, or 2% or the AMD (whichever is greater), but one or more of the quarterly determinations exceeds nine, or 2% of the AMD;

OR

The average number of medical records delinquent due to the absence of an operative report, based on at least four (quarterly) determinations is fewer than nine, or 2% of the AMOP (whichever is greater), but one or more of the quarterly determinations exceeds nine, or 2% of the AMOP.

SCORE 3 The average number of delinquent records, based on at least four (quarterly) determinations, is between 50% and 75% of the AMD, and no more than one of the determinations exceeds 100% of the AMD.

OR

The average number of medical records that are delinquent due to the absence of a medical history and physical examination, based on at least four (quarterly) determinations, exceeds nine, or 2% of the AMD (whichever is greater).

OR

The average number of medical records delinquent due to the absence of an operative report, based on at least four (quarterly) determinations, exceeds nine, or 2% of the AMOP (whichever is greater).

SCORE 4 The average number of delinquent records, based on at least four (quarterly) determinations, is between 75% and 100% of the AMD, or more than one of the quarterly determinations exceeds 100% of the AMD.

SCORE 5 The average number of delinquent records, based on at least four (quarterly) determinations, is greater than 100% of the AMD.

Note: *If the average number of delinquent medical records is greater than or equal to twice the AMD, a decision of conditional accreditation will be recommended.*

■ Standards

IM.7.8

A 1 2 3 4 5 NA   Verbal orders of authorized individuals are accepted and transcribed by qualified personnel who are identified by title or category in the medical staff rules and regulations.

IM.7.8.1

A 1 2 3 4 5 NA   Verbal orders for medications are accepted only by personnel so designated in the medical staff rules and regulations and are authenticated by the prescribing practitioner within the stated period of time.

IM.7.8.2

A 1 2 3 4 5 NA   The medical staff defines any category of diagnostic or therapeutic verbal orders associated with any potential hazard to the patient.

IM.7.8.2.1

A 1 2 3 4 5 NA   Such verbal orders are authenticated by the practitioner responsible for the patient within a time frame defined in the medical staff rules and regulations.

■ Intent of IM.7.8 Through IM.7.8.2.1

Verbal orders are frequently used in patient care. Therefore, care quality may be adversely affected if there is no mechanism designed for receiving, transcribing, and authenticating verbal orders. An appropriate mechanism is designed to

- identify qualified personnel authorized to receive the orders;
- identify certain verbal orders associated with a potential hazard to patients; and
- authenticate such verbal orders within a time frame defined in medical staff rules and regulations.

Applicable state law is considered when the time frame is established. **Note:** *For IM.7.8.2, if the medical staff has not defined any categories of diagnostic or therapeutic verbal orders associated with any potential hazard to the patient, it will be assumed that all verbal orders fall into this category and must be authenticated as defined in IM.7.8.2.1.*

■ Examples of Evidence of Performance—IM.7.8 Through IM.7.8.2.1

- Departmental policies and procedures (for example, nursing, pharmacy)
- Medical staff rules and regulations
- Review of medical records from all care sites and all clinical services provided by the organization, including records of discharged patients and patients currently in the hospital or receiving ambulatory services
- Interviews with clinical and information-management staff

■ Scoring for IM.7.8

SCORE 1 The medical staff designates in its rules and regulations who is qualified to accept verbal orders, and these rules and regulations are enforced.

SCORE 3 The medical staff designates in its rules and regulations who is qualified to accept verbal orders; however, these rules and regulations are not enforced.

SCORE 5 The medical staff does not designate in its rules and regulations who is qualified to accept verbal orders.

■ Scoring for IM.7.8.1

SCORE 1 The medical staff designates in its rules and regulations who is qualified to accept verbal orders for medications, and these rules and regulations are enforced.
AND

91% to 100% of medical records reviewed indicate that medication orders are authenticated within the time frame defined in medical staff rules and regulations.

SCORE 2 The medical staff designates in its rules and regulations who is qualified to accept verbal orders for medications, and with a few, minor exceptions, these rules and regulations are enforced.

OR

76% to 90% of medical records reviewed indicate that medication orders are authenticated within the time frame defined in medical staff rules and regulations.

SCORE 3 The medical staff designates in its rules and regulations who is qualified to accept verbal orders for medications; however, these rules and regulations are not consistently enforced.

OR

51% to 75% of medical records reviewed indicate that medication orders are authenticated within the time frame defined in medical staff rules and regulations.

SCORE 4 The medical staff designates in its rules and regulations who is qualified to accept verbal orders for medications; however, these rules and regulations are seldom enforced.

OR

26% to 50% of medical records reviewed indicate that medication orders are authenticated within the time frame defined in medical staff rules and regulations.

SCORE 5 The medical staff does not designate in its rules and regulations who is qualified to accept verbal orders for medications.

OR

Fewer than 26% of medical records reviewed indicate that medication orders are authenticated within the time frame defined in medical staff rules and regulations.

■ Scoring for IM.7.8.2

SCORE 1 Evidence indicates that the medical staff has defined any category of diagnostic or therapeutic verbal orders associated with any potential hazard to the patient.

SCORE 5 Evidence indicates that the medical staff has not defined any category of diagnostic or therapeutic verbal orders associated with any potential hazard to the patient.

■ Scoring for IM.7.8.2.1

SCORE 1 In 91% to 100% of medical records reviewed, verbal orders associated with potential hazards to the patient were authenticated within the time frame defined in the the medical staff rules and regulations.

SCORE 2 In 76% to 90% of medical records reviewed, verbal orders associated with potential hazards to the patient were authenticated within the time frame defined in the medical staff rules and regulations.

SCORE 3 In 51% to 75% of medical records reviewed, verbal orders associated with potential hazards to the patient were authenticated within the time frame defined in the medical staff rules and regulations.

SCORE 4 In 26% to 50% of medical records reviewed, verbal orders associated with potential hazards to the patient were authenticated within the time frame defined in the medical staff rules and regulations.

SCORE 5   In fewer than 26% of medical records reviewed, verbal orders associated with potential hazards to the patient were authenticated within the time frame defined in the medical staff rules and regulations.

■ Standards

IM.7.9

A 1 2 3 4 5 NA   All entries in medical records are dated and authenticated, and a method is established to identify the authors of entries.

IM.7.9.1

A 1 2 3 4 5 NA   Authentication may be by written signatures or initials, rubber-stamp signatures, or computer key.

IM.7.9.2

A 1 2 3 4 5 NA   When rubber-stamp signatures or computer key are authorized, the individual whose signature the stamp represents or whose computer key is authorized signs a statement that he or she alone will use the stamp or the code for the computer key. This statement is filed in the organization's administrative offices.

IM.7.9.2.1

A 1 2 3 4 5 NA   Such a stamp or code for the computer key is not used by another individual.

IM.7.9.3

A 1 2 3 4 5 NA   The appropriate practitioner authenticates the parts of the medical record for which he or she is responsible.

■ Intent of IM.7.9 Through IM.7.9.3

The organization has a system in place to limit access to medical records to only those authorized to make entries into the record; to identify the authors of all entries in the medical record; and to enable authors to authenticate that their entries are correct. When members of the house staff are involved in patient care, the medical record documents sufficient evidence to substantiate the active participation in, and supervision of, the patient's care by the attending physician responsible for the patient. Any entries in the medical records by house staff or nonphysicians that require countersigning by supervisory or attending medical staff members are defined in the medical staff rules and regulations.

■ Examples of Evidence of Performance— IM.7.9 Through IM.7.9.3

- Departmental policies and procedures
- Medical staff rules and regulations
- Review of medical records from all care sites and all clinical services provided by the organization, including records of discharged patients and patients currently in the hospital or receiving ambulatory services
- Interviews with clinical and information-management staff
- Demonstration of computerized patient-information systems

■ Scoring for IM.7.9

SCORE 1   In 91% to 100% of medical records reviewed, all entries identify the author and are dated and authenticated.

AND

All entries made by house staff or nonphysicians (as defined in medical staff rules and regulations) are countersigned by the appropriate supervisory or attending medical staff members.

SCORE 2	In 76% to 90% of medical records reviewed, all entries identify the author and are dated and authenticated.
SCORE 3	In 51% to 75% of medical records reviewed, all entries identify the author and are dated and authenticated.
SCORE 4	In 26% to 50% of medical records reviewed, all entries identify the author and are dated and authenticated.
SCORE 5	In fewer than 26% of medical records reviewed, all entries identify the author and are dated and authenticated.

▇ Scoring for IM.7.9.1

SCORE 1	Evidence indicates that the organization follows or uses processes, mechanisms, or policies addressing authentication methods.
SCORE 3	Evidence indicates that the organization has processes, mechanisms, or policies addressing authentication methods; however, they are not consistently followed or used.
SCORE 5	Evidence indicates that the organization does not have processes, mechanisms, or policies addressing authentication methods.

▇ Scoring for IM.7.9.2

SCORE 1   The organization has a mechanism designed to ensure the security of the identification method used by the practitioner to authenticate records. This mechanism requires a signed statement by the individual authorized to use a rubber-stamp signature or code for computer key.
AND
The statement is filed in the organization's administrative offices.

SCORE 5 The organization does not have a mechanism designed to ensure the security of the identification method used by the practitioner to authenticate records.

■ Scoring for IM.7.9.2.1

SCORE 1 The rubber-stamp signature or computer key is used only by the authorized individual.

SCORE 5 The rubber-stamp signature or computer key is used by someone other than the authorized individual.

■ Scoring for IM.7.9.3

SCORE 1 In 91% to 100% of medical records reviewed, the appropriate practitioner has authenticated the parts of the record for which he or she is responsible.

SCORE 2 In 76% to 90% of medical records reviewed, the appropriate practitioner has authenticated the parts of the record for which he or she is responsible.

SCORE 3 In 51% to 75% of medical records reviewed, the appropriate practitioner has authenticated the parts of the record for which he or she is responsible.

SCORE 4 In 26% to 50% of medical records reviewed, the appropriate practitioner has authenticated the parts of the record for which he or she is responsible.

SCORE 5 In fewer than 26% of medical records reviewed, the appropriate practitioner has authenticated the parts of the record for which he or she is responsible.

■ Standards

IM.7.10

A 1 2 3 4 5 NA   When a patient is admitted to the hospital or appears for a pre-scheduled ambulatory care appointment, the organization uses a patient information system to routinely assemble all divergently located record components. The system also ensures that all record components are assembled in a timely manner, as needed for patients seen for unscheduled ambulatory and emergency services visits.

IM.7.10.1

A 1 2 3 4 5 NA   The medical record or computer system indicates when a portion of the record has been filed elsewhere to alert authorized personnel of the portion's existence.

■ Intent of IM.7.10 and IM.7.10.1

Practitioners have on hand or have ready access to any relevant information about any care the patient may have previously received anywhere in the organization, including its ambulatory care service or its emergency service. This applies if the patient is admitted to the hospital or is seen for a prescheduled ambulatory care visit, as well as for an unscheduled outpatient visit or an emergency service visit. Such information facilitates continuity of care among multiple providers and over time for a single provider. This information is provided in a timely manner by hard copy or screen display.

■ Examples of Implementation— IM.7.10 Through IM.7.10.1

1. Using the unit record is one way to effectively combine records of care generated by different departments or subdivisions of the organization. The same purpose can be served

by inserting ambulatory care and emergency care records in the inpatient record at the time of an inpatient admission. An alternative approach is to insert significant material, such as the discharge resume, operative notes, and pathology reports, from the inpatient record into the ambulatory care and emergency care records.

2. A computer-based patient record can assemble information about the patient that is stored in multiple databases in the organization.
3. A protocol for what is requested by discipline and physician is developed, and this information is then provided to the practitioner in a timely manner.

■ Examples of Evidence of Performance— IM.7.10 Through IM.7.10.1

- Departmental policies and procedures
- Medical staff rules and regulations
- Interviews with clinical and information-management staff
- Demonstration of computerized patient-information systems

■ Scoring for IM.7.10

SCORE 1 In 91% to 100% of medical records reviewed, all the patient's relevant requested inpatient, ambulatory care, and emergency care records were assembled manually or electronically when the patient received care.

SCORE 2 In 76% to 90% of medical records reviewed, all the patient's relevant requested inpatient, ambulatory care, and emergency care records were assembled manually or electronically when the patient received care.

SCORE 3 In 51% to 75% of medical records reviewed, all the patient's relevant requested inpatient, ambulatory care, and emergency care records were assembled manually or electronically when the patient received care.

SCORE 4 In 26% to 50% of medical records reviewed, all the patient's relevant requested inpatient, ambulatory care, and emergency care records were assembled manually or electronically when the patient received care.

SCORE 5 In fewer than 26% of medical records reviewed, all the patient's relevant requested inpatient, ambulatory care, and emergency care records were assembled manually or electronically when the patient received care.

∎ Scoring for IM.7.10.1

SCORE 1 The medical record or computer system indicates when a portion of the record is filed elsewhere.
AND
This portion of the medical record can be retrieved easily whenever the practitioner needs it.

SCORE 2 With a few, minor exceptions, the medical record or computer system indicates when a portion of the record is filed elsewhere.
AND
With a few, minor exceptions, this portion of the medical record can be retrieved easily whenever the practitioner needs it.

SCORE 3 The medical record or computer system does not consistently indicate when a portion of the record is filed elsewhere.
OR

This portion of the medical record cannot consistently be retrieved easily whenever the practitioner needs it.

SCORE 4 The medical record or computer system seldom indicates when a portion of the record is filed elsewhere.
OR
This portion of the medical record can seldom be retrieved easily whenever the practitioner needs it.

SCORE 5 The medical record or computer system does not indicate when a portion of the record is elsewhere.
OR
This portion of the medical record cannot be retrieved easily whenever the practitioner needs it.

EXHIBIT 6 Aggregation Summary

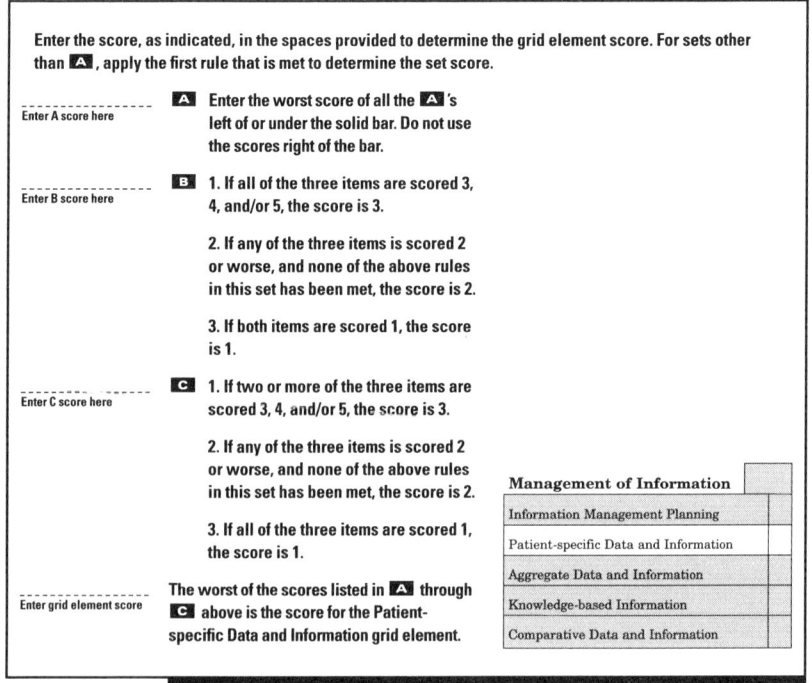

Aggregate Data and Information

■ Standards

IM.8

A 1 2 3 4 5 NA The information-management function provides for the definition, capture, analysis, transmission, and reporting of data and information that can be aggregated to support managerial decisions and operations, performance-improvement activities, and patient care.

IM.8.1 *Data and information that can be aggregated include at least the following:*

IM.8.1.1

A 1 2 3 4 5 NA Pharmacy transactions as required by applicable law and as necessary to adequately control and account for all drugs, including:

IM.8.1.1.1

A 1 2 3 4 5 NA Maintaining a means of identifying the signatures of all practitioners authorized to prescribe or order medications; and

IM.8.1.1.2

A 1 2 3 4 5 NA A listing of practitioners' Drug Enforcement Administration numbers, where required.

IM.8.1.2 *Information about hazards and safety practices used to identify safety management issues to be addressed by the safety committee, including:*

IM.8.1.2.1

A 1 2 3 4 5 NA Summaries of the deficiencies, problems, failures, and user errors in safety management, life safety management, equipment management, and utilities management, as well as relevant published reports of hazards associated with any of these areas;

IM.8.1.2.2

A 1 2 3 4 5 NA Documented surveys, at least semiannually, of all areas of the facility to identify environmental hazards and unsafe practices; and

IM.8.1.2.3

A 1 2 3 4 5 NA Reports and investigations of all incidents involving property damage, occupational illness, or patient, personnel, or visitor injury.

IM.8.1.3

A 1 2 3 4 5 NA Records of radionuclides and radiopharmaceuticals, including the radionuclide's identity, the date received, method of receipt, activity, recipient's identity, date administered, and disposal;

IM.8.1.4

A 1 2 3 4 5 NA Records of any required reporting to proper authorities;

IM.8.1.5

A 1 2 3 4 5 NA A coding and retrieval system for medical records by diagnosis and procedure;

IM.8.1.6

A 1 2 3 4 5 NA A coding and retrieval system for patient demographic information;

IM.8.1.6.1

A 1 2 3 4 5 NA A continuously maintained control register for emergency and outpatient services* includes at least the following information for every individual seeking care: identification, such as name, age, and sex; date, time, and means of arrival; nature of complaint; disposition; and time of departure.

IM.8.1.7

A 1 2 3 4 5 NA A coding and retrieval system for financial information;

IM.8.1.8

A 1 2 3 4 5 NA Measures (that is, indicators) of processes and outcomes for assessing performance;

IM.8.1.9

A 1 2 3 4 5 NA Summaries of actions taken as the result of organizationwide performance-improvement activities, including risk management, utilization review, infection control, and safety management;

IM.8.1.10

A 1 2 3 4 5 NA Practitioner-specific information for licensed independent practitioners, as defined in the "Medical Staff" chapter of the *CAMH*;

IM.8.1.11

A 1 2 3 4 5 NA The ability to gather accurate, timely information for both operational decision making and planning purposes; and

---

* **Outpatient services** refers to a patient appointment system, and all the requirements in the standard do not apply.

IM.8.1.12

A 1 2 3 4 5 NA Data and information to support clinical research, as desired.

■ Intent of IM.8 Through IM.8.1.12

Clinical and administrative data can be aggregated and analyzed for supporting decisions, tracking trends over time, making comparisons within the organization and among organizations, and improving performance.

■ Example of Implementation—IM.8 Through IM.8.1.12

Aggregate information can be collected from large numbers of medical records to support clinical research. For instance, the organization can aggregate data from patients with similar problems and analyze the results of various treatment options to determine efficacy. Other examples of patient data that may be aggregated to improve performance are data for blood usage review, surgical case review, and drug usage evaluation. Examples of data and information that may require tracking for reporting purposes are birth and death registration, transfusion-related fatalities, contagious diseases, adverse drug reactions, immunizations, abuse victims, gunshot wounds, reports to the Food and Drug Administration and/or the manufacturer of a medical device-related death or serious injury or illness caused or contributed to by that device; and any required records for adequate control and accountability for medical devices.

■ Examples of Evidence of Performance—IM.8 Through IM.8.1.12

- Information-management policies and procedures
- Reports of aggregate data and information
- Interviews with clinical and information-management staff

■ Scoring for IM.8

SCORE 1   Evidence indicates that the organization assesses its needs for aggregate data and information in managerial decisions and operations, performance-improvement activities, and patient care.

SCORE 2   With a few, minor exceptions, evidence indicates that the organization assesses its needs for aggregate data and information in managerial decisions and operations, performance-improvement activities, and patient care.

SCORE 3   Evidence indicates that the organization does not consistently assess its needs for aggregate data and information in managerial decisions and operations, performance-improvement activities, and patient care.

SCORE 4   Evidence indicates that the organization seldom assesses its needs for aggregate data and information in managerial decisions and operations, performance-improvement activities, and patient care.

OR

Evidence indicates that the organization does not assess its needs for aggregate data and information in performance-improvement activities, or patient care.

SCORE 5   Evidence indicates that the organization does not assess its needs for aggregate data and information in managerial decisions and operations, performance-improvement activities, and patient care.

■ Scoring for IM.8.1

This standard is not scored.

Scoring for IM.8.1.1

SCORE 1 The organization has a mechanism in place designed to maintain control and accountability of all drugs in the pharmacy.

SCORE 3 The organization has a mechanism in place designed to maintain control and accountability of all drugs in the pharmacy, but it is not consistently enforced.

SCORE 5 The organization does not have a mechanism in place designed to maintain control and accountability of all drugs in the pharmacy.

Scoring for IM.8.1.1.1

SCORE 1 The organization maintains a means of identifying the signatures of all practitioners authorized to prescribe or order medications.

SCORE 3 The organization does not consistently maintain a means of identifying the signatures of all practitioners authorized to prescribe or order medications.

SCORE 5 The organization does not maintain a means of identifying the signatures of all practitioners authorized to prescribe or order medications.

Scoring for IM.8.1.1.2

SCORE 1 There is a listing of practitioners' Drug Enforcement Administration numbers, where required.

SCORE 5 There is no listing of practitioners' Drug Enforcement Administration numbers, where required.

Scoring for IM.8.1.2
This standard is not scored.

■ Scoring for IM.8.1.2.1

SCORE 1 The organization uses a system for collecting and processing aggregate safety information for safety management, life safety management, equipment management, and utilities management for use by the safety committee and other appropriate individuals.

SCORE 2 With a few, minor exceptions, the organization uses a system for collecting and processing aggregate safety information for the areas listed in Score 1 for use by the safety committee and other appropriate individuals.

SCORE 3 The organization uses a system for collecting aggregate safety information for the areas listed in Score 1, but this information is not processed for use by the safety committee and other appropriate individuals.

SCORE 4 The organization uses a system for collecting aggregate safety information for the areas listed in Score 1, but this information is not collected from a variety of sources.
AND
This information is not processed for use by the safety committee and other appropriate individuals.

SCORE 5 The organization does not use a system for collecting and processing aggregate safety information for the areas listed in Score 1 for use by the safety committee and other appropriate individuals.

■ Scoring for IM.8.1.2.2

SCORE 1 The organization uses a system for collecting and processing aggregate safety information from surveys of all the facility's areas to identify environmental hazards and unsafe practices for use by the safety committee and other appropriate individuals, as specified in the "Management of the Environment of Care" chapter of the *CAMH*.

SCORE 2 With a few, minor exceptions, the organization uses a system for collecting and processing aggregate safety information from surveys of all the facility's areas to identify environmental hazards and unsafe practices for use by the safety committee and other appropriate individuals, as specified in the "Management of the Environment of Care" chapter of the *CAMH*.

SCORE 3 The organization uses a system for collecting aggregate safety information from surveys of all the facility's areas to identify environmental hazards and unsafe practices, but this information is not processed for use by the safety committee and other appropriate individuals, as specified in the "Management of the, Environment of Care" chapter of the *CAMH*.

SCORE 4 The organization uses a system for collecting aggregate safety information, but the information is not collected from safety surveys as described in Score 1.
AND
The information is not processed for use by the safety committee and other appropriate individuals, as specified in the "Management of the Environment of Care" chapter of the *CAMH*.

SCORE 5 The organization does not use a system for collecting and processing aggregate safety information from surveys of all the facility's areas to identify environmental hazards and unsafe practices for use by the safety committee and other appropriate individuals, as specified in the "Management of the Environment of Care" chapter of the *CAMH*.

■ Scoring for IM.8.1.2.3

SCORE 1 The organization uses a system for collecting and processing aggregate safety information from reports and investigations of all incidents involving property damage, occupational illness, or patient, personnel, or visitor injury for use by the safety committee and other appropriate individuals.

SCORE 2 With a few, minor exceptions, the organization uses a system for collecting and processing aggregate safety information from the sources listed in Score 1 for use by the safety committee and other appropriate individuals.

SCORE 3 The organization uses a system for collecting aggregate safety information from the sources listed in Score 1, but this information is not processed for use by the safety committee and other appropriate individuals.

SCORE 4 The organization uses a system for collecting aggregate safety information, but this information is not collected from sources listed in Score 1.
AND
The information is not processed for use by the safety committee and other appropriate individuals.

SCORE 5 The organization does not use a system for collecting and processing aggregate safety information from the sources listed in Score 1 for use by the safety committee and other appropriate individuals.

■ Scoring for IM.8.1.3

SCORE 1   The organization maintains detailed records for the receipt, use, and disposal of radionuclides and radiopharmaceuticals.

SCORE 2   With a few, minor exceptions, the organization maintains detailed records for the receipt, use, and disposal of radionuclides and radiopharmaceuticals.

SCORE 3   The organization does not consistently maintain detailed records for the receipt, use, and disposal of radionuclides and radiopharmaceuticals.

SCORE 4   The organization seldom maintains detailed records for the receipt, use, and disposal of radionuclides and radiopharmaceuticals.

SCORE 5   The organization does not maintain detailed records for the receipt, use, and disposal of radionuclides and radiopharmaceuticals.

■ Scoring for IM.8.1.4

SCORE 1   The organization uses a system to collect aggregate data and information from appropriate sources regarding records of any required reporting to proper authorities for use in managerial decisions and operations, performance-improvement processes, and patient care.

SCORE 2   With a few, minor exceptions, the organization uses a system to collect aggregate data and information from appropriate sources regarding records of any required reporting to proper authorities for use in managerial decisions and operations, performance-improvement processes, and patient care.

SCORE 3	The organization does not consistently use a system to collect aggregate data and information from appropriate sources regarding records of any required reporting to proper authorities for use in managerial decisions and operations, performance-improvement processes, and patient care.
SCORE 4	The organization seldom uses a system to collect aggregate data and information from appropriate sources regarding records of any required reporting to proper authorities for use in managerial decisions and operations, performance-improvement processes, and patient care.
SCORE 5	The organization does not use a system to collect aggregate data and information from appropriate sources regarding records of any required reporting to proper authorities for use in managerial decisions and operations, performance-improvement processes, and patient care.

■ Scoring for IM.8.1.5

SCORE 1	The organization uses a coding and retrieval system to collect aggregate data and information from appropriate sources for medical records by diagnosis and procedure for use in managerial decisions and operations, performance-improvement processes, and patient care.
SCORE 2	With a few, minor exceptions, the organization uses a coding and retrieval system to collect aggregate data and information from appropriate sources for medical records by diagnosis and procedure for use in managerial decisions and operations, performance-improvement processes, and patient care.

SCORE 3 The organization inconsistently uses a coding and retrieval system to collect aggregate data and information from appropriate sources for medical records by diagnosis and procedure for use in managerial decisions and operations, performance-improvement processes, and patient care.

SCORE 4 The organization seldom uses a coding and retrieval system to collect aggregate data and information from appropriate sources for medical records by diagnosis and procedure for use in managerial decisions and operations, performance-improvement processes, and patient care.

SCORE 5 The organization does not use a coding and retrieval system to collect aggregate data and information from appropriate sources for medical records by diagnosis and procedure for use in managerial decisions and operations, performance-improvement processes, and patient care.

Scoring for IM.8.1.6

SCORE 1 The organization uses a coding and retrieval system to collect aggregate patient demographic data and information from appropriate sources for use in managerial decisions and operations, performance-improvement processes, and patient care.

SCORE 2 With a few, minor exceptions, the organization uses a coding and retrieval system to collect aggregate patient demographic data and information from appropriate sources for use in managerial decisions and operations, performance-improvement processes, and patient care.

SCORE 3 The organization inconsistently uses a coding and retrieval system to collect aggregate patient demographic data and information from appropriate sources for use in managerial decisions and operations, performance-improvement processes, and patient care.

SCORE 4 The organization seldom uses a coding and retrieval system to collect aggregate patient demographic data and information from appropriate sources for use in managerial decisions and operations, performance-improvement processes, and patient care.

SCORE 5 The organization does not use a coding and retrieval system to collect aggregate patient demographic data and information from appropriate sources for use in managerial decisions and operations, performance-improvement processes, and patient care.

■ Scoring for IM.8.1.6.1

SCORE 1 The organization uses a system to collect aggregate information from a continuously maintained control register for emergency services that includes the following information for every individual seeking care: identification, such as name, age, and sex; date, time, and means of arrival; nature of complaint; disposition; and time of departure.
AND
The organization maintains an appointment system for outpatient services.

SCORE 2 The organization uses a system to collect aggregate information from a continuously maintained control register for emergency services that includes seven or eight of the items listed in Score 1.

SCORE 3 The organization uses a system to collect aggregate information from a continuously maintained control register for emergency services that includes five or six of the items listed in Score 1.

AND

The organization does not maintain an appointment system for outpatient services.

SCORE 4 The organization uses a system to collect aggregate information from a continuously maintained control register for emergency services that includes three or four of the items listed in Score 1.

SCORE 5 The organization uses a system to collect aggregate information from a continuously maintained control register for emergency services that includes fewer than three of the items listed in Score 1.

OR

The organization does not use a system to collect aggregate information from a continuously maintained control register for emergency services and a system for appointment for outpatient services.

Scoring for IM.8.1.7

SCORE 1 The organization uses a coding and retrieval system to collect aggregate financial data and information from appropriate sources for use in managerial decisions and operations, performance-improvement processes, and patient care.

SCORE 2 With a few, minor exceptions, the organization uses a coding and retrieval system to collect aggregate financial data and information from appropriate sources for use in managerial decisions and operations, performance-improvement processes, and patient care.

SCORE 3   The organization inconsistently uses a coding and retrieval system to collect aggregate financial data and information from appropriate sources for use in managerial decisions and operations, performance-improvement processes, and patient care.

SCORE 4   The organization seldom uses a coding and retrieval system to collect aggregate financial data and information from appropriate sources for use in managerial decisions and operations, performance-improvement processes, and patient care.

SCORE 5   The organization does not use a coding and retrieval system to collect aggregate financial data and information from appropriate sources for use in managerial decisions and operations, performance-improvement processes, and patient care.

▬ Scoring for IM.8.1.8

SCORE 1   The organization uses a system of measures (that is, indicators) to collect aggregate data and information from appropriate sources about processes and outcomes for assessing performance and for use in managerial decisions and operations, performance-improvement processes, and patient care.

SCORE 2   With a few, minor exceptions, the organization uses a system of measures (that is, indicators) to collect aggregate data and information from appropriate sources about processes and outcomes for assessing performance and for use in managerial decisions and operations, performance-improvement processes, and patient care.

SCORE 3   The organization inconsistently uses a system of measures (that is, indicators) to collect aggregate data and information from appropriate sources about processes and outcomes for assessing performance and for use in managerial decisions and operations, performance-improvement processes, and patient care.

SCORE 4 The organization seldom uses a system of measures (that is, indicators) to collect aggregate data and information from appropriate sources about processes and outcomes for assessing performance and for use in managerial decisions and operations, performance-improvement processes, and patient care.

SCORE 5 The organization does not use a system of measures (that is, indicators) to collect aggregate data and information from appropriate sources about processes and outcomes for assessing performance and for use in managerial decisions and operations, performance-improvement processes, and patient care.

■ Scoring for IM.8.1.9

SCORE 1 The organization uses a system to collect from appropriate sources summaries of actions taken as a result of organizationwide performance-improvement activities, including risk management, utilization review, infection control, and safety management. These aggregate data and information are used in managerial decisions and operations, performance-improvement processes, and patient care.

SCORE 2 With a few, minor exceptions, the organization uses a system to collect from appropriate sources summaries of actions as described in Score 1.

SCORE 3 The organization inconsistently uses a system to collect from appropriate sources summaries of actions as described in Score 1.

SCORE 4 The organization seldom uses a system to collect from appropriate sources summaries of actions as described in Score 1.

SCORE 5 The organization does not use a system to collect from appropriate sources summaries of actions as described in Score 1.

■ Scoring for IM.8.1.10

SCORE 1 The organization uses a system to collect aggregate licensed independent practitioner-specific data and information from appropriate sources for use in managerial decisions and operations, performance-improvement processes, and patient care.

SCORE 2 With a few, minor exceptions, the organization uses a system to collect aggregate licensed independent practitioner-specific data and information from appropriate sources for use in managerial decisions and operations, performance-improvement processes, and patient care.

SCORE 3 The organization inconsistently uses a system to collect aggregate licensed independent practitioner-specific data and information from appropriate sources for use in managerial decisions and operations, performance-improvement processes, and patient care.

SCORE 4 The organization seldom uses a system to collect aggregate licensed independent practitioner-specific data and information from appropriate sources for use in managerial decisions and operations, performance-improvement processes, and patient care.

SCORE 5 The organization does not use a system to collect aggregate licensed independent practitioner-specific data and information from appropriate sources for use in managerial decisions and operations, performance-improvement processes, and patient care.

■ Scoring for IM.8.1.11

SCORE 1 The organization uses a system to collect accurate, timely aggregate information from appropriate sources for both operational decision making and planning purposes.

SCORE 2 With a few, minor exceptions, the organization uses a system to collect accurate, timely aggregate information from appropriate sources for both operational decision making and planning purposes.

SCORE 3 The organization does not consistently use a system to collect accurate, timely aggregate information from appropriate sources for both operational decision making and planning purposes.

SCORE 4 The organization seldom uses a system to collect accurate, timely aggregate information from appropriate sources for both operational decision making and planning purposes.

SCORE 5 The organization does not use a system to collect accurate, timely aggregate information from appropriate sources for both operational decision making and planning purposes.

■ Scoring for IM.8.1.12

SCORE 1   The organization uses a system to collect aggregate data and information from appropriate sources to support clinical research.

SCORE 2   With a few, minor exceptions, the organization uses a system to collect aggregate data and information from appropriate sources to support clinical research.

SCORE 3   The organization does not consistently use a system to collect aggregate data and information from appropriate sources to support clinical research.

SCORE 4   The organization seldom uses a system to collect aggregate data and information from appropriate sources to support clinical research.

SCORE 5   The organization does not use a system to collect aggregate data and information from appropriate sources to support clinical research.

EXHIBIT 7   Aggregation Summary

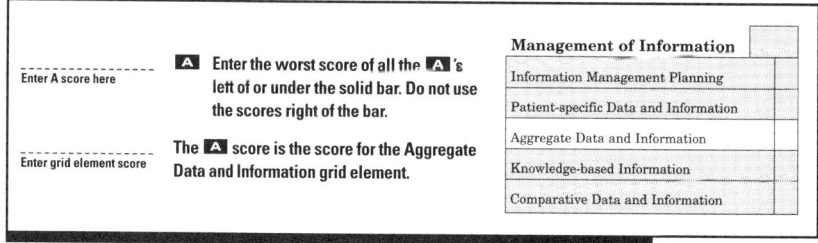

Knowledge-based Information

■ Standard

IM.9 *The management of knowledge-based information (also referred to as "literature") provides for the identification, organization, retrieval,* *analysis, delivery, and reporting of clinical and managerial journal literature, reference information, and research data for use in designing, managing, and improving patient-specific and organizational processes.*

▰ Intent of IM.9

Knowledge-based information refers to authoritative, up-to-date print and nonprint information resources, including current periodicals, indexes, and abstracts in print or electronic format; recent editions of texts and other resources; and patient education materials in response to individual and organizational needs. Knowledge-based information supports clinical and management decision making, performance-improvement activities, continuing education of staff, patient and family education, and research. All types of information do not have to be provided on site. An organization is not required to have a library located in its facility. These services may be shared with other hospitals or community resources, if a mechanism is in place designed to make needed information accessible to hospital staff in a timely manner.

▰ Scoring for IM.9

This standard is not scored.

▰ Standard

IM.9.1

A 1 2 3 4 5 NA   The organization provides systems, resources, and services to meet its informational, educational, and, when appropriate, research-related needs for knowledge-based information and literature.

▰ Intent of IM.9.1

Knowledge-based information management consists of systems, resources, and services to help health professionals acquire and maintain the knowledge and skills needed to care for patients, support clinical and management decision making, and provide needed information and education to patients and families. The organization provides mechanisms designed for acquiring, assembling, and transmitting information to users as well as the means to accomplish these objectives. The extent of services provided is based on the organization's assessed needs.

■ Example of Implementation — IM.9.1

To practice medicine effectively, physicians have access to medical knowledge bases and know how to apply this information to plan and evaluate therapies. Physicians are familiar with various types of information technology that allow them to access and manage medical information for patient care.

■ Scoring for IM.9.1

SCORE 1 Evidence indicates that the organization has a plan for and provides clinical and managerial literature, reference information, and research data to meet its identified needs (see IM.9.2).

SCORE 2 With a few, minor exceptions, evidence indicates that the organization provides the information sources listed in Score 1 to meet its identified needs.
AND
Evidence indicates that the organization has a plan (part of a larger organizational plan, a separate plan, minutes, or reports) to identify the need for and to provide clinical and managerial literature, reference information, and research data and information.

SCORE 3 Evidence indicates that the organization inconsistently provides the information sources listed in Score 1 to meet its identified needs.
OR
There is no evidence that the organization has a plan (part of a larger organizational plan, a separate plan, minutes, or reports) to identify the need for and to

provide clinical and managerial literature, reference information, and research data and information.

SCORE 4 Evidence indicates that the organization seldom provides the information sources listed in Score 1 to meet its identified needs.

SCORE 5 Evidence indicates the organization does not provide the information sources listed in Score 1 to meet its identified needs.

Standards

IM.9.2

A 1 2 3 4 5 NA The extent of knowledge-based information services, resources, and systems (for example, professional library and health information services) is related not only to the organizational services provided, but also to the needs of the medical and nursing staffs, administrators and managers, other health professional staff, other organization staff, students, patients and their families, and researchers.

IM.9.2.1 *The assessment of the organizational needs for knowledge-based information considers*

IM.9.2.1.1

A 1 2 3 4 5 NA the need for accessibility and timeliness;

IM.9.2.1.2

A 1 2 3 4 5 NA the need to link with the organization's internal information systems; and

IM.9.2.1.3

A 1 2 3 4 5 NA the need to link with appropriate external databases and information networks.

■ Intent of IM.9.2 Through IM.9.2.1.3

The organizational information needs assessment considers the need for knowledge-based information. Library and information services enable the organization to

- use knowledge-based information by responding to information requests from the clinical and management staffs, other organizational staff, and patients and their families, as appropriate;
- provide information in advance by anticipating information needs and systematically linking the literature with clinical and organizational processes; and
- provide relevant, current, and accurate information within appropriate time frames and in formats appropriate to recipients' needs.

Information is accessible in one or more of the following ways:
- Immediately at the work site;
- Within the hospital in a shared central collection (for example, a professional library); and/or
- From outside sources with acceptable time delays (for example, from vendors or other institutions).

The quality of either proactive or responsive information service can be judged by the following criteria: accuracy, currency, relevance to the request, speed of response, format (ease of use), and validity of the information.

■ Examples of Evidence of Performance— IM.9.2 Through IM.9.2.1.3

- Written plans
- Surveys of needs
- Meeting minutes

■ Scoring for IM.9.2

SCORE 1 Evidence indicates that the needs assessment is used in planning the services, resources, and systems of knowledge-based information.

| SCORE 2 | Evidence indicates that, with a few, minor exceptions, the needs assessment is used in planning the services, resources, and systems of knowledge-based information. |

| SCORE 3 | Evidence indicates that the needs assessment is not consistently used in planning the services, resources, and systems of knowledge-based information. |

| SCORE 4 | Evidence indicates that the needs assessment is seldom used in planning the services, resources, and systems of knowledge-based information. |

| SCORE 5 | Evidence indicates that the needs assessment is not used in planning the services, resources, and systems of knowledge-based information. |

■ Scoring for IM.9.2.1

This standard is not scored.

■ Scoring for IM.9.2.1.1 Through IM.9.2.1.3

Note: *The following set of scoring guidelines applies to standards IM.9.2.1.1 through IM.9.2.1.3. The checkmark at Score 2 applies to IM.9.2.1.2 and IM.9.2.1.3. The checkmark at Score 3 applies to IM.9.2.1.1.*

| SCORE 1 | Evidence indicates that the needs for knowledge-based information are assessed and the relevant factor identified in the standard is taken into account. |

| SCORE 2 | Evidence indicates that the needs for knowledge-based information are assessed and, with a few, minor exceptions, the relevant factor identified in the standard is taken into account. |

| SCORE 3 | Evidence indicates that the needs for knowledge-based information are assessed; however, the relevant factor identified in the standard is not consistently taken into account. |

SCORE 4 Evidence indicates that the needs for knowledge-based information are assessed; however, the relevant factor identified in the standard is seldom taken into account.

SCORE 5 Evidence indicates that the needs for knowledge-based information are not assessed.

▄ Standard

IM.9.3

A 1 2 3 4 5 NA Systems and structures (electronic or paper based) provide for the appropriate identification, organization, retrieval, analysis, delivery, and reporting of knowledge-based information and literature to meet identified needs.

▄ Intent of IM.9.3

Electronic or paper-based systems and structures (often in the form of professional library services) organize knowledge-based information resources and facilitate the provision of information services. Systems and structures are in place for organizing, locating, using, and sharing the organization's knowledge-based information and literature. Systems and structures are also in place for identifying (subject access), retrieving, and delivering knowledge-based information and literature. Systems and structures provide appropriate controls to assure uniformity, completeness, and compatibility with bibliographic and other records.

▄ Example of Implementation—IM.9.3

An organization's information system may include automated or paper catalogs organized by author, title, journal, and subject, or simply provide the location of sources of information and other lists of resources. Examples of electronic or paper-based systems and structures that facilitate identification of knowledge-based information include subject indexes (for example, Index Medicus, Medline), systems that provide access to medical and university libraries at the international, national, regional, and local levels. Systems and structures for locating and delivering appropriate information include networks providing access to other library holdings, clearinghouses, commercial information services, and international, national, regional, and local systems for sharing resources (for example, the British Library, the National Library of Medicine, local consortia). Examples of controls are subject thesauri (for example, Medical Subject Headings); classification systems (the National Library of Medicine Classification System); the Marc format for bibliographic description; agreements, regulations, policies, and procedures for cooperative resource sharing; and codes for interlibrary lending (for example, the Interlibrary Loan code of the American Library Association).

■ Scoring for IM.9.3

SCORE 1 Evidence indicates that there are systems and structures for organizing books, journals, and other resources (for example, catalogs, on-line databases); subject access to internal and external resources (for example, subject catalogs, indexes, and on-line or CD-ROM bibliographic databases); and delivering needed information resources not owned by the organization (for example, reciprocal sharing agreements, consortia membership).

SCORE 2 Evidence indicates that, with a few, minor exceptions, there are systems and structures that fulfill all three functions identified in Score 1.

SCORE 3 Evidence indicates that there are systems and structures that fulfill only two of the three functions identified in Score 1.

SCORE 4 Evidence indicates that there are systems and structures that fulfill only one of the three functions identified in Score 1.

SCORE 5 Evidence indicates that there are no systems and structures that fulfill any of the three functions identified in Score 1.

■ Standards

IM.9.4

A 1 2 3 4 5 NA Accessible knowledge-based information resources include clinical and management literature (in appropriate formats, including paper or electronic journals, books, technical reports, and audiovisuals); externally produced databases; practice guidelines; and information in multiple formats for patient education (brochures, articles, pamphlets, audiovisual materials, and models).

IM.9.4.1

A 1 2 3 4 5 NA The organization's knowledge-based information resources are authoritative and up to date.

■ Intent of IM.9.4 and IM.9.4.1

Knowledge-based resources are accessible to everyone in the organization who needs them. These resources provide authoritative and up-to-date scientific, clinical, and managerial knowledge. Examples of authoritative resources include reference materials, such as *Selected List of Books and Journals for the Small Medical Library* (referred to as the Brandon-Hill list), published every other year by the Medical Library Association (MLA) in the *Bulletin of the MLA;* and the *Library for Internists,* published by the American College of Physicians every three years in the *Annals of Internal Medicine.* Other methods of selecting authoritative, up-to-date resources include scanning databases and publishing information, following customer recommendations, and using reviews.

■ Scoring for IM.9.4

SCORE 1 Evidence indicates that knowledge-based information resources are available to everyone who needs them.

SCORE 2 Evidence indicates that, with a few, minor exceptions, knowledge-based information resources are available to everyone who needs them.

SCORE 3 Evidence indicates that knowledge-based information resources are not consistently available to everyone who needs them.

SCORE 4 Evidence indicates that knowledge-based information resources are seldom available to everyone who needs them.

SCORE 5 Evidence indicates that knowledge-based information resources are not available to everyone who needs them.

■ Scoring for IM.9.4.1

SCORE 1 Evidence indicates that knowledge-based information resources are authoritative and up to date.

SCORE 2 Evidence indicates that, with a few, minor exceptions, knowledge-based information resources are authoritative and up to date.

SCORE 3 Evidence indicates that knowledge-based information resources are not consistently authoritative and up to date.

SCORE 4 Evidence indicates that knowledge-based information resources are seldom authoritative and up to date.

SCORE 5 Evidence indicates that knowledge-based information resources are not authoritative and up to date.

■ Standards

IM.9.5

A 1 2 3 4 5 NA The pharmacy, medical, and nursing staff has access to poison-control information.

IM.9.6

A 1 2 3 4 5 NA A hospital formulary or drug list is readily available to the staff who use it.

■ Intent of IM.9.5 and IM.9.6

Poison-control and formulary information are readily available. A poison-control center hotline is usually the most effective, up-to-date source of information.

■ Scoring for IM.9.5

SCORE 1 The organization has ready access to current poison-control information for emergency reference.

SCORE 5 The organization does not have ready access to current poison-control information for emergency reference.

■ Scoring for IM.9.6

SCORE 1 Formulary or drug list information is current and available for those who use it.

SCORE 3 Formulary or drug list information is current but not consistently available for those who use it.

SCORE 5 No formulary or drug list is available in the organization.

EXHIBIT 8 Aggregation Summary

		Management of Information	
------------------ Enter A score here	**A** Enter the worst score of all the **A**'s left of or under the solid bar. Do not use the scores right of the bar.	Information Management Planning	
		Patient-specific Data and Information	
------------------ Enter grid element score	The **A** score is the score for the Knowledge-based Information grid element.	Aggregate Data and Information	
		Knowledge-based Information	
		Comparative Data and Information	

Comparative Data and Information

■ Standards

IM.10 *The information-management function provides for the definition, capture, analysis, transmission, and reporting and/or use of comparative performance data and information, the comparability of which is based on national and state guidelines for data set parity and connectivity.*

IM.10.1

A 1 2 3 4 5 NA The organization uses external reference databases for comparative purposes.

IM.10.2

A 1 2 3 4 5 NA The organization contributes to external reference databases when required by law or regulation and/or when appropriate to the organization.

IM.10.3

A 1 2 3 4 5 NA The information-management function maintains the security and confidentiality of data and information when contributing to or using external databases.

■ Intent of IM.10 Through IM.10.3

The organization uses external data and information to identify deviations from expected patterns or trends and also contributes information to external reference databases, as required or appropriate, such as the Joint Commission Indicator Measurement System (IMSystem) database and national or regional registries. The information-management function provides for the exchange of clinical and knowledge-based data and information with other health care organizations, when appropriate and feasible. The intent of these standards is to develop the organization's future capabilities and goals.

■ Examples of Implementation— IM.10 Through IM.10.3

1. A "reference" database provides useful feedback for evaluating the performance of organizations contributing data to the database. Reference databases fall into one or more of the following categories:
   - Multihospital System Databases—These databases can be voluntary or mandatory and can include a few hospitals in a local system or hundreds of hospitals nationally. The content of each database varies. Sponsors of these types of databases include the Daughters of Charity, Hospital Corporation of America, Voluntary Hospitals of America, the Department of Veterans Affairs, and the Department of Defense.
   - Disease- or Diagnosis-Specific Databases—These databases are primarily patient oriented and include, for example, trauma registries, cancer registries, databases regarding arthritis, AIDS, hemophilia, or any particular discharge DRG.
   - Procedure-Specific Databases—These databases are primarily related to patient care procedures (possibly captured in procedure codes) and include, for example, those related to coronary artery bypass graft, prosthetic valve replacement, artificial joint replacement, ophthalmology lens implantation, and so forth.
   - Management Databases—Frequently operated by state hospital associations, these include, for example, data on

financial performance, staffing, safety, equipment, and similar operational factors. Some examples include the Connecticut Health Information Management and Exchange (CHIME) database and the Commission on Professional and Hospital Activities (CPHA).

- Investigational Databases—These databases are supported most frequently by larger health care organizations that conduct research and can include databases related to a drug protocol, treatment choice or protocol, or a particular device or technical procedure.
- Proprietary Databases—Some of these databases are maintained by firms that develop and market "risk adjustment" software to hospitals. MediQual Inc.'s "MedisGroups" database is well known, but there are numerous others such as Iameter, Inc., Computerized Severity of Illness Index (CSI), and Systemetric's Coded Disease Staging. Private firms, such as Lexecon, Inc. (Chicago) and HCIA, Inc. (Baltimore) among many others, also collect clinical, financial, marketing, and other data, and prepare comparative reports for their clients.
- Quality Improvement Databases—Some databases have been developed specifically to provide participants with comparative information on health care processes and outcomes. Examples include the Joint Commission's Indicator Measurement System (IMSystem) and the Maryland Hospital Association's Quality Improvement (QI) Project. Quality improvement networks and consortiums also may sponsor such databases for their members.
- Purchase/Payer Databases—Projects such as the Greater Cleveland Quality Health Choice Project, a collaborative effort of major employers and hospitals, may establish and operate reference databases for their members. Similar efforts are underway in other areas.
- State Agency Databases—More states are mandating hospital participation in data collection and submission.

Not all agencies currently provide comparative feedback, but many do, such as Illinois Cost Containment Council and the Pennsylvania Health Care Cost Containment Council.

Many databases are very comprehensive and can serve multiple purposes, such as for understanding costs related to a particular treatment choice for a particular diagnosis.

2. Comparative information from reference databases on processes and/or patient outcomes help organizations set priorities for improving performance and provide benchmarking information about improvement opportunities. Sources of comparative information include state hospital associations for printouts of information (financial, staffing efficiency studies); professional organizations; the Maryland Hospital Association Quality Indicator Project; cancer database (tumor registry); and the Joint Commission's IMSystem. Within a large multihospital system (such as the Department of Defense or the Department of Veterans Affairs) encompassing many similar hospitals, a database containing data from hospitals within the system permits each hospital to compare itself to other system hospitals.

Examples of Evidence of Performance— IM.10.1 Through IM.10.3

- Organizationwide policies and procedures
- Departmental policies and procedures
- Interviews with the organization's leaders and staff
- Agreements with reference database(s) for access and/or participation

Scoring for IM.10

This standard is not scored.

Scoring for IM.10.1

SCORE 1   The organization uses external reference databases for comparative purposes.

SCORE 2 The organization is starting to implement a plan to use external reference databases for comparative purposes.

SCORE 3 The organization has a plan to use external reference databases for comparative purposes but has not started to implement it.

SCORE 5 The organization does not use comparative data from external reference databases and does not have a plan to do so.

■ Scoring for IM.10.2

SCORE 1 The organization provides information to at least one external reference database from which it can obtain comparative data.

SCORE 2 The organization is starting to implement a plan to contribute to external reference databases from which it can obtain comparative data.

SCORE 3 The organization has a plan to contribute to external reference databases from which it can obtain comparative data, but it has not started to implement it.

SCORE 5 The organization does not provide information to at least one external reference database from which it can obtain comparative data.

■ Scoring for IM.10.3

SCORE 1 The security and confidentiality of data and information are maintained when contributing to or using an external reference database.

SCORE 2 Note: *Although the surveyor will score this standard at an organization's actual level of performance, the impact of the score will be no greater than a Score 2.*

SCORE 3 The organization has a plan to assure appropriate security and confidentiality of data and information when contributing to or using an external reference database but has not started to implement it.

SCORE 5 The security and confidentiality of data and information are not maintained when contributing to or using an external reference database.

EXHIBIT 9 Aggregation Summary

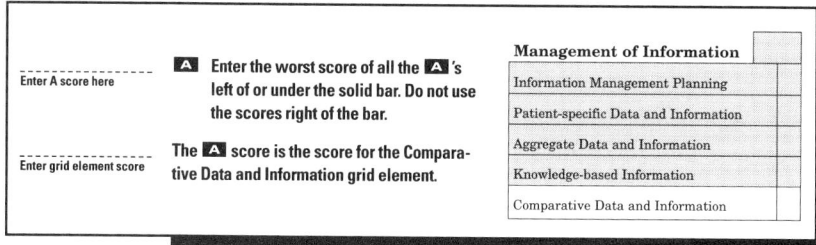

SUGGESTED READINGS AND OTHER RESOURCES

Dick RS, Steen EB (eds): *The Computer-Based Patient Record: An Essential Technology for Health Care.* Institute of Medicine. Washington, D.C.: National Academy Press, 1991.

Advocates the development and implementation of computer-based patient records (CPRs). Discusses the current state of patient record systems, presents the basic components of future CPRs, and outlines a plan for widespread CPR implementation.

Fuchs B: Translating data into information: A primer of preparatory concepts and skills. *Top Health Rec Manage* 12(4): 25–32, 1992.

Outlines the steps involved in establishing a data plan. Discusses the concepts and skills necessary for translating data into information.

Gabrieli ER: Aspects of a computer-based patient record. *J AHIMA* 64(7): 70–82, 1993.

Probes the history, development, and future potential of computer-based patient records. Discusses the growing interest in computer-based health care records, the contents and structure of paper charts and the retrieval of those records, the retrievability of on-line patient records, the tools for electronic patient record generation, the need for standardization, accessing the data in computer-processed patient records, and problems with computer-based patient records.

Gostin LO, et al: Privacy and security of personal information in a new health care system. *JAMA* 270(20): 2487–2493, 1993.

Examines the privacy and security goals for the collection, storage and use of health care information in a new health care system and the means to attain those goals. Discusses the ethical framework for privacy and the nature of patient rights issues relating to the collection and release of data.

Huffman EK: *Medical Record Management*, 10th ed. Berwyn, IL: Physicians Records Co, 1994.

Outlines the basic concepts of medical record science, including development and content of hospital medical records, management of content and storage, classification systems, indexes and registers, health care statistics, information systems in health care, and medical records in ambulatory care, long-term care, and rehabilitation facilities.

Quality control for medical transcription. *J Am Assoc Med Transcr* 13(1): 14, 1994.

Contains recommended guidelines by the American Association for Medical Transcription for adequate quality control for medical transcription.

APPENDIX B

An Overview of the Joint Commission's Indicator Measurement System

The Joint Commission's Indicator Measurement System (IMSystem) is an indicator-based performance measurement system designed to help health care organizations measure and improve their performance and to assist the Joint Commission in evaluating the performance of health care organizations as part of the survey and accreditation process.

The IMSystem includes 31 indicators in 1995 related to obstetrical, perioperative, and oncology care; 7 indicators for cardiovascular care; and 9 indicators related to trauma care. Indicator development was led by expert task forces; each indicator's relevancy, reliability, and validity were assessed through long-term processes. In 1996, the Joint Commission plans to add measures related to medication use and infection control.

Organizations that participate in the IMSystem continuously collect data elements used for the indicators and periodically submit them to the Joint Commission's national repository. The Joint Commission aggregates and analyzes these performance data to provide individualized comparative reports.

A key factor related to an organization's participation in the IMSystem is the successful integration of performance measurement data elements into its existing automated data-gathering environment. Recognizing the already tremendous information burdens on most organizations, the Joint Commission has designed the IMSystem to be parsimonious (that is, to collect only those data elements that are needed and to use all the elements that are collected). Whenever possible, the IMSystem uses data elements likely to be already collected by health care organizations.

■ Technology Requirements

The IMSystem data elements and requirements for automated data collection and submission to the Joint Commission are detailed in the Joint Commission's *Software Specifications* manual. Indicator field testing was supported by the development of related data collection and submission software. While the Joint Commission has delineated the requirements for participating in the IMSystem, health care organizations have several options for meeting these requirements:

- Organizations that maintain their own information systems may choose to incorporate the functions described in the *Software Specifications* manual into their existing systems to permit collection of the required data elements.
- Organizations supported by outside vendors may request that software changes be made by their vendors to accommodate the IMSystem data collection requirements. The specifications manual has been made available to all information system vendors free of charge.
- Organizations may purchase and install a stand-alone data collection software package. Several vendors have developed PC-based stand-alone software products to support the IMSystem. The Joint Commission is providing the *Software Specifications* manual to all information system developers and vendors free of charge. The IMSystem Help Desk maintains a vendor contact list identifying companies who have contacted the Joint

Commission about developing IMSystem software solutions. The 3M Health Care's PC-product "3M IMSystem" has been tested and endorsed by the Joint Commission as one solution to facilitate participation in the IMSystem. Other products may best meet the needs of some participants.

The alternatives listed above allow health care organizations the freedom to choose the solution that best meets their needs, while supporting an efficient data collection process. Organizations requiring additional information on technology options may contact the IMSystem help desk at (708) 916-5220. Regardless of the method selected for implementation, the resulting system should be able to

- collect reliable and accurate data;
- generate reports that identify missing data needed;
- accurately calculate indicator categories for each episode of care;
- generate reports to assist with interpreting and using indicator data;
- prepare and create data files in the proper format necessary for submission to the Joint Commission's indicator data repository;
- submit the indicator data to the IMSystem in an electronic, machine-readable format such as modem file transfer, diskette, or tape;
- reconcile errors or discrepancies and resubmit specific episode-of-care records for correction processing; and
- perform maintenance and utility functions.

■ Use of IMSystem Data

In the future, performance measures will be used by the Joint Commission to enhance the survey and accreditation process. The IMSystem and other databases will provide information to both the Joint Commission and the accredited organization about the organization's ongoing performance between triennial on-site surveys. Measurement results, *per se,* will not necessarily determine accreditation status. Rather, trends and patterns of indicator rates may trigger a response from the Joint Commission to assess an organization's use of the indicator data to improve performance, its compliance with standards in areas that affect the indicator rates, and/or the possible need for education or other assistance. The use of indicator data in the focusing of on-site accreditation surveys is also being determined. Participation in an outcomes measurement system such as the IMSystem is expected to be required when system data are used in evaluation activities associated with accreditation. This is not likely to occur before 1997.

It is anticipated that organizations will use indicator data not only to discover ways to improve services, but also to better understand their *processes* of care, to identify problems with current processes, and to manage risk. Organizations also can use the IMSystem to respond to requests for performance data, a likely scenario under health care reform. Finally, payers, purchasers, patients, and researchers will use indicator data to choose providers, to clarify policy options, to initiate regulatory evaluations, and to study the health care system and the efficacy of treatment.

▰ Participation

Beginning in 1994, the Joint Commission invited optional participation in the IMSystem by hospitals only. Participants are subject to specific terms of agreement.

To facilitate participation and system implementation by hospitals, wherever possible, the Joint Commission promotes system efficiencies by working through hospital associations, multi-hospital systems, and/or information system vendors. Potential cooperative arrangements include:

- Participating hospitals forward indicator data to the partner organization (association, alliance, system, or vendor), which pools the data for its own analysis and performs a single transmission to the Joint Commission's database;
- Participating hospitals forward their data directly to the Joint Commission's database and authorize the Joint

Commission to release their data to the partner organization for state- or system-level comparative analyses or other value-added services;
- Participating hospitals forward their data directly to the Joint Commission's database and authorize the Joint Commission to develop state- or system-level comparative reports, which are provided to the partner organization for use in consultation, education, or other value-added services for the participating institutions.

In all cases, the partner organization works with the Joint Commission staff to provide information to its member hospitals about the value of involvement in the IMSystem and to meet the education and training needs of the enrolling institutions.

■ Confidentiality

Once outcome measurement data are integrated into survey and accreditation activities, organization-specific data may be released to respond to the growing public demand for data on quality and performance of health care organizations. Until that time, however, organization-specific IMSystem data will be considered confidential and will not be voluntarily disclosed by the Joint Commission. Neither will Joint Commission surveyors receive organization-specific IMSystem data for use in survey and accreditation activities, unless provided to the surveyors by the participating organization. Organization-specific IMSystem data, which is collected after outcome measures become integral to the accreditation process, may be subject to the Joint Commission's Confidentiality and Disclosure Policy found in the *Accreditation Manual for Hospitals*. At that time, such data will be used by surveyors in on-site survey activities.

The IMSystem is intended to provide information that can be used by health care organizations to assess and improve their services, by the Joint Commission to monitor and guide performance improvement in accredited organizations, and by the public in making decisions about their own health care.

APPENDIX C

Additional Resources

■ Complying with Joint Commission Standards

Brandt M: New Joint Commission standards: Management of information roles of health information management professionals. *Journal of AHIMA* 64(11):81–84, Nov 1993.

The author outlines the significant challenges associated with implementing the Joint Commission's new management of information standards. She argues that, for many, the requirements will be difficult to meet; but "integration of existing databases is critical to the development of the nationwide computer-based patient record required for health care in the 21st century."

Corum W: JCAHO standards and systems integration. *Healthcare Informatics* 11:22–28, Jan 1994.

New management of information standards for health care networks address issues not covered in existing accreditation manuals, including "networkwide integration, coordination, and accountability." The author points out that information systems must include more than what currently exists, and he discusses the need for strategic planning. System integration benefits are also covered, including an example of how one hospital was able to perform the same procedure with the same result as another hospital for 75% less cost.

Roberts CR: What can you expect during your on-site survey? *Journal of AHIMA* 65(4):66–69, Apr 1994.

A good explanation of the Joint Commission's "new team approach" to surveys is provided. The author explains what to expect during the survey and includes a sample survey agenda. She also gives examples of what questions may be asked of staff (for example, nursing, dietary, health information) and provides some advice on how to prepare for a survey, as well as what to do following the survey.

Thomason M: Implementing the Joint Commission standards: One hospital's approach. *Journal of AHIMA* 65(5):66–69, May 1994.

This article gives an excellent review of how one health care organization has prepared and organized for compliance with the Joint Commission's management of information requirements. Much dedication and hard work have paid off for the organization. For example, the organization volunteered for a test survey by the Joint Commission. Details of what staff had to resolve and how it was done are covered. Sample forms that help define objectives and strategic planning are also included.

Information Planning

Davenport TH: Saving IT's soul: Human-centered information management. *Harv Bus Rev* 72:119–131, Mar/Apr 1994.

Davenport stresses that people handle information. He points out that glorifying information technology and ignoring human psychology can be a disaster. To have an effective information system, the author explains that "management must begin by thinking about how people use information—not with how people use machines." "The Information Facts of Life" are outlined and discussed. Examples from several corporations are covered, including the problems they faced and their solutions. The author warns "we must abandon the idea that technology in and of itself can solve a company's information problems."

Hopkins JL: An information strategy to improve and measure quality. *QRC Adviser* 9(2):1–6, Dec 1992.

To meet the demands of the future, the author believes a radically different approach to information management is needed. There are reasons for sharing information to develop quality care throughout an organization. Since prevailing systems are driven by financial data, the future must be driven by clinical data. Possible objections are covered, and valid reasons given for rethinking the design of information systems for quality improvement.

Iguanzo JM, Pol L: Building the data intensive hospital. *Hospitals and Health Networks* 67:80, Oct 1993.

The authors stress the importance of data that staff members can access and apply both to broad issues, such as strategic planning and to the solution of day-to-day problems. The article stresses that staff members need to understand the need for and purpose and use of data.

Krueger Wilson C: Quality-driven information systems: A time to act. *J Nurs Care Qual* 7(1):7–15, Oct 1992.

In this era, where the focus is on the cost and quality of health care services, the author finds it difficult to believe that "professional nursing has not been able to effectively apply information technology in order to document nursing outcomes." Effective information systems will be the basis for quality health care, and for successful compliance with new standards. As the author states, "The design and implementation of quality driven information systems is not an impossibility. However, it takes significant commitment, a major shift in thinking, adequate resources, and specialized knowledge." Much is discussed relative to the inadequacy of most present day systems, but the article gives counsel for the attainment of a quality program.

Roberts C: Developing an information management plan. *Journal of AHIMA* 65(5):19–23, May 1994.

Roberts stresses that health information-management professionals should definitely be involved in the development of a facility's information-management plan. She gives the whys and hows for writing such a plan. To begin, she suggests bringing a crossfunctional team together, including the hospital administrator, chief information officer, directors of admitting, patient accounts, nursing, and so forth. She concludes that a good plan is a major project, but it can be accomplished if taken in small increments.

Spath PL: The interface of quality management and the hospital information department. *Top Health Inform Manage* 13(3):1–11, Feb 1993.

The author describes how quality management activities are "dependent upon valid and reliable data about health care processes and patient outcomes." The paper then illustrates how information-management professionals can use continuous quality improvement techniques to meet this challenge. By identifying their primary customers and understanding those customers' needs and expectations, health information departments can begin to design appropriate systems that support quality management activities.

Stall M, et al: Long-range planning for information systems. *Healthcare Financial Management* 46(6):36–46, Jun 1992.

Although developing a long-range plan for information systems might appear to be an overwhelming task, the authors claim it can be a simple exercise for a community hospital. They cover the planning process appropriate for community health care providers, including why a plan should be created, who should participate, planning objectives, data gathering, information system objectives, current information environment, findings and recommendations, investment requirements, and action plan. Exhibits outlining the phases are included.

Stodolak F, Carr J: Systems must be compatible with quality efforts. *Healthcare Financial Management* 46(6):72–77, Jun 1992.

The data needed to pursue total quality management and/or continuous quality improvement are incomplete and/or inconsistent, the author argues. Involvement of managers and employees from all disciplines within the hospital is a requirement for successful quality efforts. Thus, there is need for a common database manager. This, and creating the same language, will allow individuals from one department to load information from another department onto their personal computers without having to learn a new system. Exhibits covering database management software are provided, and advantages of common database managers are explained. Suggestions to get started are also included.

■ Training

Wager KA: Herbert RR: Using a hospital information system in the classroom environment. *Top Health Inform Manage* 13(4):83–89, May 1993.

Both authors are associated with the educational program for Health Information Administration at the Medical University of South Carolina Medical Center. This article summarizes much of the background and activity that occurred in introducing students to information systems with state-of-the-art technology in the classroom.

Parmalee JC: Achieving empowerment through information. *Top Health Inform Manage* 13(4):15–29, May 1993.

With a new computer system, the Albany Medical Center has been able to set up "a source of reliable, consistent, integrated data with which to set goals, monitor performance, and make decisions." The article provides a before-and-after scenario.

■ Case Studies

Aldridge GK, et al: Managing the implementation of a pharmacy information system. *Am J Hosp Pharm* 50:1198–1203, Jun 1993.

The author argues that "the implementation of a new computerized information system is a major challenge that is increasingly confronting pharmacists." This article provides a full explanation of what is involved in implementing a pharmacy information system, including the preimplementation and discussions with other departments, the "construction" phase, the "delivery," the "implementation," and the postimplementation. This provides an idea of how to implement, even when an existing system exists.

Barnhart DM: Scripps Clinic: In transition to the on-line medical record. *J Ambulatory Care Manage* 15(3):1–12, Jul 1992.

Scripps Clinic's Transcription Mainframe Interface project (TMI) is described in some detail as it relates to the clinic's strategic information plan, which was nearing completion at the time this article was written. The project's history and goals are outlined, including the selection of vendors and how staff evaluated the product, as well as what was required for the system. A year after the TMI system was implemented at the Scripps campus, physicians "are accessing lab results and documents from home via modem to review the next day's patients or while on call."

Bennett JJ, et al: A computer-based patient record: Emory's approach. *Top Health Inform Manage* 13(4):51–62, May 1993.

In 1991, the Emory University System of Health Care began to automate its medical record. The article describes Emory's reasons for developing a computer-based patient record (CPR) and factors that are attributed to its success, including a commitment of chief executives, vendor partnerships, project organization, a progressive approach, clinician participation, a well-planned pilot, and a focus on training and support.

Harris C, Conner CB: Building a computer-supported quality improvement system in one year: The experience of a large state psychiatric hospital. *The Joint Commission Journal on Quality Improvement* 20(6):330–342, Jun 1994.

To attain Joint Commission accreditation, a large state psychiatric hospital implemented a data-intensive quality improvement (QI) program. This article is a good description of how a quality improvement program was established by using available statistical software. The authors say, "If we could have developed this statistical software-based QI in only one year, then virtually any organization, large or small, can attain the technical capability to conduct state-of-the-art QI."

Minard B, et al: Reengineering and improving the information-intensive work of patient tracking for inpatients and outpatients. *Top Health Inform Manage* 14(3):7–20, Feb 1994.

During the 1980s, The Methodist Hospital's (Houston) concentration on continuous quality improvement (CQI) resulted in innovative systems and procedures. These innovations included: removal of department boundaries, unified booking and registration of patients, system capabilities for patient reservations, patient movement improvements, decentralized room management functions, precise recording of the locations of patients, and more. "We are now implementing our plan to move record keeping to the point of care, near and at patients' bedsides, and using computer terminals that are portable and can be moved to or carried into patients rooms."

Teague DK, Laraia MT: Success factors for automated systems in the clinical environment: The MUSC experience. *Top Health Inform Manage* 14(3):21–28, Feb 1994.

In the hope of changing "the current state of inefficient automated clinical information systems," the Medical University of South Carolina and Bell Atlantic Healthcare Systems prepared for the successful testing and implementation of the Open Architecture Clinical Information System (OACIS). This article provides several details on how a carefully implemented plan was put into operation.

Weiss KM, Chapman HA: Computer-assisted inpatient psychiatric assessment and treatment planning system. *Hospital and Community Psychiatry* 44:1097–1100, 1993.

Why is a computer-assisted treatment plan useful? The authors explain that, with a single document, it provides a record that clearly specifies the patient's symptoms on admission, and how the patient responded to treatment over time. It focuses the treatment team's attention on specific target symptoms, rather than on global categories. It creates and provides access to a database that can be used to examine characteristics of hospitalized patients both cross-sectionally and longitudinally.

▄ Medical Records

Barnett GO, Jenders RA, Chueh HC: The computer-based clinical record—where do we stand? *Annals of Internal Medicine* 119:1046–1048, 1993.

Authors state that a "major impediment to the development of a computer-based clinical record system has been the lack of agreement in standards both for the clinical terminology to be used and for the computer technology." For computer-based records systems to be maximally effective, they must completely replace the paper record. To achieve this adaptation, it requires the "modification of longstanding traditions of medical record keeping." The authors report on the collaboration of Health Level Seven with the American Society for Testing and Materials (ASTM), and their efforts to implement a standard for the protocol to be used in the communication of laboratory data in an electronic format. They believe the absence of vocabulary standards has led to noncompatible systems and programs. The lack of standards makes it difficult to properly measure treatment cost-effectiveness, and to learn how patient outcomes are affected by clinical decisions.

England SP: One positive impact of health care reform to physicians: The computer-based patient record. *Top Health Inform Manage* 14(2):38–47, Feb 1993.

Mr. England's final statement is "Hence, health system reengineering must begin and be developed where health information is initially created—in the physician's office or clinic." This is preceded with reasons for health care reform and its requirements. The author argues that the shift by government regulators and third-party payers from "cost control" to "outcome management control" requirements could "cave the system in." He says that the time has come to focus on a complete restructuring of the U.S. health care system "in terms of how it is financed, delivered, and managed." He believes all physicians will be faced with computer-based patient records (CPR). Community-based systems and their benefits to physicians and managed health care networks are covered. In addition, cost savings and estimated costs to develop and implement a CPR are explained.

Fletcher DM: The system analysis as a tool for medical record department improvements. *Journal of AHIMA* 62(12):38–46, Dec 1991.

The author is the director of the medical record department at HCA Wesley Medical Center in Wichita, Kansas. The article provides a step-by-step examination of her department's quality improvement efforts. The article is an excellent review and detailed explanation of how a large 760-bed medical center improved its medical record department. This improvement was in conjunction with, and compatible with improvements being attained by, the medical center itself.

Gabrieli ER: Aspects of a computer-based patient record. *Journal of AHIMA* 64(7): 70–82, Jul 1993.

This piece probes the history, development, and future potential for computer-based patient records. It discusses the growing interest in computer-based health care records, the medical contents of a paper chart and retrieval of those records, the retrievability of on-line patient records, the structure of information in a traditional patient chart, the tools for electronic patient record generation (input of dictated or written notes, automated medical test analyzer, structure of medical facts, encoding, databanks), the need for standardization (for longitudinal compatibility, comparability, compressibility, standard nomenclature), accessing the data in computer-processed patient records, and problems with computer-based patient records (the need for new skills, the input of data, the output of data, special procedures to ensure confidentiality).

General Accounting Office (GAO), Committee of Governmental Affairs, U.S. Senate: *Automated medical records: Leadership Needed to Expedite Standards Development.* Washington, DC: GAO, April 1993.

Although electronic sharing of medical data is crucial to the effective and efficient delivery of quality health care, more than a decade of effort has yielded little agreement among public and private interests on the standards required to develop an automated medical records system. As a result, U.S. health care practitioners continue to rely on a cumbersome, paper-based clinical records system that has remained largely unchanged for decades. Efforts to develop automated medical record standards have been stymied by a lack of leadership. Several voluntary organizations have been most active in developing standards. But the complex nature of medical care, the large number of standards needed, and the variety of special interests involved in standards development have made this a daunting task. To date, the federal role in this effort has been limited. GAO believes that more active federal involvement could speed standards development.

Johnson G: Computer-based patient record systems—A planned evolution. *Healthcare Informatics* 11:43–51, Jan 1994.

Acknowledging that there are several ways computer-based patient records can be implemented, the author describes common steps in all these approaches, which include automating and integrating, information retrieval by clinician, functions for information entry, integrating institutions at the community level, and tying communities together into a national network. "Healthcare reform is moving to the top of the country's political agenda, and CPR systems are viewed as a major part of the solution to improve quality and reduce costs."

Martin CA: Improving the quality of medical record documentation. *Journal of Healthcare Quality* 14(3):16–23, May–Jun 1992.

The author describes the efforts of one hospital to revise and upgrade its medical record documentation by means of quality improvement strategies. She stresses that accurate and complete medical record documentation is essential in any health care setting. In addition to communicating vital patient care information, the medical record provides documentation of appropriate evaluation, treatment, and services. It also is used to evaluate practitioner performance, to monitor resource use, and to determine reimbursement.

Whiting-O'Keefe EQ, et al: A computerized summary medical record system can provide more information than the standard medical record. *JAMA* 25:1185–1192, 1985.

The Summary Time-Oriented Record (STOR), a computerized outpatient medical record system, is assessed for its ability to communicate information to clinicians. The authors report the results of two randomized single-blind studies: (1) When STOR was added to the standard medical record, it was found that physicians were better able to predict their patients' future symptoms than when the standard medical record was used. Also, this applied to laboratory results from outpatient visits. (2) In a separate study, the removal of the standard medical record did not result in any important decrease in the physician's ability to predict patients' symptoms, as well as laboratory test results (that is, if they had the option of 514 visits, the physicians exercised this option). The article concludes that, for outpatient visits, the STOR operationally added information that was supplied by the full-paper medical record. This improved flow of information could improve the clinical decision process.

■ Confidentiality and Security

Drislane D: Keeping medical records private in the electronic information age. *Journal of American Health Policy* 4:28–32, Mar/Apr 1994.

The author compares confidentiality mechanisms in current paper-based systems with those in electronic information systems. The many reasons why an electronic system will create an environment that will be more secure, as well as help in providing better medical care quality, are detailed. How a security policy and information technology can protect patient medical data is illustrated in an example of a computerized system developed by Harvard Community Health Plan's Clinic. The author suggests a national policy that outlines what constitutes an invasion of confidentiality, what type of information should be protected and to what degree, what constitutes authorized access and use, who is accountable for ensuring the integrity of the system, and what penalties should be instituted for violation.

Gostin LO, et al: Privacy and security of personal information in a new health care system. *JAMA* 270(20):2487–2493, Nov 1993.

This article examines the privacy and security goals for the collection, storage, and use of health care information in a new health care system and the means to attain those goals. The goals are: (1) to ensure the integrity of the health care data; (2) to ensure the availability of health data for authorized persons; and (3) to ensure the privacy of patients relative to the disclosure of information. It discusses the ethical framework for privacy as well as the nature of patient rights issues relating to the collection and release of data that should be addressed within the dialogue of informed consent. It is recommended that there be involvement within the organization in the context of ethics and data management.

■ Data

Torchia M: Using data to improve quality. *Business & Health* 12:23–27, Mar 1994.

Employers are finding that there are many advantages to being equipped with specific data on the performance of their health care plans. These benefits include cost controls and better health care for their employees. Three employers are featured with examples of what they have and hope to accomplish by analyzing claims and utilizing data. Since each company had distinct characteristics, the examples show common, yet separate, solutions to problems in handling their managed health care system for their employees (for example, vendor surveillance, overutilization, and measuring cost effectiveness).

■ Knowledge-Based Information

Lindberg DAB, et al: Use of MEDLINE by physicians for clinical problem solving. *JAMA* 269(24):3124–3129, Jun 1993.

"MEDLINE is a bibliographic database containing more than 7 million citations, most with abstracts, from over 3,500 biomedical journals and covering the period 1966 to present." The National Library of Medicine (NLM) initiated a study to find the full range of situations, and results of using this on-line database. This article chronicles the complete study. It goes into the design, the methods, the participants, and so forth. It was found that information obtained from MEDLINE had an impact on clinical problem solving, choosing the appropriate diagnostic tests, making the diagnosis, and more. The authors, in their conclusion, indicate it was found that MEDLINE was used for a diversity of needs. "There were even reported instances in which the information obtained via a MEDLINE search was critical to saving a patient's life."

Medical Library Association (MLA): Standards for Hospital Libraries, 1994 ed. Chicago: MLA, 1994.

These standards "are intended to provide medical librarians and administrators with a definition of library and information services, and to provide opportunities and challenges for developing enhanced library services in health care institutions." The Medical Library Association standards focus on the importance of management of information to the delivery of quality health care.

■ Hardware and Software Decisions

Abdelhak Mervat, et al: Hospital information systems applications and potential: A literature review revisited, 1982–1992. *Top Health Inform Manage* 13(4): 1–14, May 1993.

Many developments have occurred from 1982 to 1992 in the diffusion and application of information systems in health care institutions. The article includes the evolution of administrative applications, but the majority of articles reviewed focus on clinical applications (for example, computer-assisted diagnosis systems, systems to teach diagnostic skills, video programs for patient teaching, systems for ambulatory care, and more). The necessary issues to be addressed are confidentiality, security, legality, and standardization.

Kibbe DC, Scoville RP: Computer software for healthcare CQI. *Quality Management in Health Care* 1(4):50–58, Summer 1993.

The article describes the data and information demands that will result from the transition from traditional quality assurance (QA) to continuous quality improvement (CQI). The authors hope to help "health care leaders visualize the role for personal computer technology in CQI implementation." They demonstrate the difference between centralized and decentralized data management. They examine the new role for information services under CQI and what software to consider. Based on experience, the authors give several suggestions to help in selection (for example, ease of learning, flexibility, analytical capabilities).

Ventura MR, et al: Selecting and using computer application software for quality assessment and improvement. *J Nurs Care Qual* 7(1):16–28, Oct 1992.

The advantages of using computer applications programs over manual methods is stressed for quality assessment and improvement (QAI). First, the authors give a guide for the selection of a computer system, which includes four steps (that is, need, comparison, selection, and compatibility). The following question is posed: "Will using computer technology allow an individual to process work more efficiently, and enable the individual to do things that were not possible manually?" Guides for selecting a computer system and software systems are detailed.

■ Information Networks

Gardner E: Shared information could revolutionize healthcare. *Modern Healthcare* Vol:30–36, Oct 1992.

"Think of it: claims, outcomes, patient records, administrative costs on one system as a resource for all providers and payers in a network." This article gives thoughts on the future, where there could be annual savings of $4 billion to $10 billion, if health care transactions were conducted electronically. The author describes the differences between "community health networks" and "community health *information* networks." She also lists some communities and statewide networks that are operating, testing, or planning systems, including New York State's demonstration project. Costs, confidentiality concerns, and other challenges are covered.

Special issue of *Health Progress:* Plugging into the future: Integrated information systems, April 1994.

1. Vital links for today and tomorrow. This is a success story of an information-management system implemented by Provident Health Partners (PHP) in Denver. The integrated delivery system network includes three Denver area hospitals and several outpatient facilities. Benefits have included decreases in operating costs, improvement in quality hospital performance, and an increase in patient loyalty. Proposed future uses are discussed.

2. "Rural Connections." Details the inadequacies inherent in rural health care delivery and why the belief that fiber-optic technology may be the answer to these problems. Also, the article summarizes how two multi-institutional providers with 27 hospitals in Iowa are conferring with state and federal representatives on the possibilities of joining an existing statewide communication system and/or possible federal funding for development of telemedicine applications.

3. Building a patient record system. This article gives some ideas relative to the computerized patient record (CPR) concept for the future. It outlines Genesy Health System's (Flint, Michigan) plans to "build out continuum of care into a regional integrated healthcare delivery system." The authors contend that the development of a CPR precedes a regional integrated health care delivery system. There are many benefits summarized as well as the importance of reliability in input. Health care executives are advised to examine their business and clinical issues to determine their desires or needs.

Lumsdon K, et al: The clinical connection. Hospitals work to design information systems that physicians will use. *Hospitals* 67:16–26, May 1993.

A series of short case studies illustrate the variety of ways that health care organizations are integrating information technology into clinical settings. Issues covered include the computer's introduction to the clinical setting, the development of automated clinical protocols and decision-support systems, and the emergence of computer networks linking hospitals' and physicians' practices. Organizations from across the country are profiled.

■ Book Titles of Interest

Ball MJ, et al: *Healthcare Information Management Systems.* New York: Springer-Verlag, 1991.

Dick RS, Steen EB: *The Computer-Based Patient Record: An Essential Technology for Health Care.* Institute of Medicine. Washington, DC: National Academy Press, 1991.

Huffman EK: *Medical Record Management,* 9th ed. Berwyn, IL: Physicians Records Co, 1990.

Orthner JF, Blum BI: *Implementing Health Care Information Systems.* New York: Springer-Verlag, 1989.

Worthley JA, Disalvio PS: *Managing Computers in Health Care,* 2nd ed. Health Administration Press, 1989.

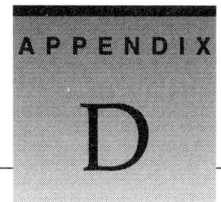

APPENDIX D

Management of Information Terms

Aggregate: To combine standardized data and information.

Assess: To transform data into information by analyzing the data.

Authenticate: To provide authorship, for example, by written signature, identifiable initials, or computer key.

Bias: An effect tending to product results that depart systematically from the true value (to be distinguished from random error).

Clinical resume: A component of the medical record consisting of concise recapitulation of the reasons for hospitalization, the significant findings, the procedures performed, the treatment rendered, the condition of the patient on discharge, and any specific instructions given to the patient and/or family.

Confidentiality: Safekeeping of data and information as restricted to individuals who have need, reason, and permission for access to such data and information.

Data: Uninterpreted observations or facts.

Data capture: The acquisition or recording of data and information.

Data connectivity: The ability to link data.

Data definition: The identification of the data to be used in analysis.

Data integrity: The accuracy, consistency, and completeness of data.

Data parity: The equivalency of data.

Database: A collection of stored data.

Function: A group of activities and processes with a common goal.

Information: An interpreted set(s) of data; organized data that provide a basis for decision making.

Knowledge-based information: A collection of stored facts, models, and information that can be used for designing and redesigning processes and for problem solving. In the context of the AMH, knowledge-based information is found in the clinical, scientific, and management literature.

Medical record: The account compiled by physicians and other health care professionals of a variety of patient health information, such as the patient's assessment findings, treatment details, and progress notes.

Medical records, complete: A medical record is complete when: (1) its contents reflect the diagnosis, results of diagnostic tests, therapy rendered, condition and in-hospital progress of the patient, and condition of the patient at discharge; and (2) its content, including any required clinical resume or final progress notes are assembled and authenticated, and all final diagnoses and any complications are recorded without the use of symbols or abbreviations.

Minimum data set: An agreed-upon and accepted set of terms and definitions constituting a core set of data; a collection of related data items.

Performance measure: A measure, such as a standard or indicator, used to assess the performance of a function or process of any organization.

Quality of documentation: The degree to which information recorded in source documents is accurate and complete and is performed in a timely manner.

Security: The protection of data from intentional or unintentional destruction, modification, or disclosure.

Transformation: The process of changing the form of data representation, for example, changing data into information with the use of decision analysis tools.

Transmission: The sending of data and information from one location to another.

Validity: Verification of correctness.

Other General Definitions

Collection: Information collected and aggregated.

Integration: Data generated must be mixed and interrelated.

Analysis: Trends, patterns, and variation identified; creates context.

Reporting: Communicate information in a way that is meaningful for decision making; information is stripped of complexity and "techno-gab."

Sources

Beckham, J. Daniel: The approach of the number crunchers. *Healthcare Forum Journal* 35:71–74, Sep/Oct 1992.

Joint Commission: 1995 *Accreditation Manual for Hospitals.* Oakbrook Terrace, IL: Joint Commission, 1994.

APPENDIX E

Sample Information Management Plan

The following information-management plan was developed by Mecosta County General Hospital, Big Rapids, Michigan, with the assistance of First Consulting Group, Pittsburgh, Pennsylvania. It is presented solely to illustrate an approach to the management of information and to stimulate readers' thoughts on the subject. As noted in Chapter 2, the Joint Commission does not require an information-management plan. An information-management plan may constitute evidence of compliance with IM.1: "Information-management processes are planned and designed to meet the health care organization's internal and external information needs." However, meeting minutes, various types of reports, and other documentation may also be used to document these planning activities. (See Chapter 2, "Planning for the Management of Information," page 23, for more on this.)

Mecosta County General Hospital
Big Rapids, Michigan

INFORMATION SYSTEM STRATEGY SUMMARY

■ I. Mission and Philosophy

I-1. Role: This strategy specifies the role that information technology should play in supporting strategic business goal attainment.
- Use information technology selectively to enhance quality and/or operating efficiency with the primary focus on operational requirements and management control.

I-2. Image: This strategy specifies how information technology should be deployed to influence how the hospital is to be perceived by patients, employees, physicians, the community, and other external groups.
- Desire to move quickly to implement new technologies after they have been tested by the industry and pricing has been stabilized.

I-3. Risk: This strategy specifies the relative level of risk to which the management team is willing to expose the hospital regarding the acquisition and implementation of information systems and related technologies.
- Willing to assume some risks in high priority areas, but with solid confidence in an ability to manage inherent risks.

I-4. Cost: This strategy specifies the hospital's ability and willingness to invest in formation system acquisition and operation.
- Balance investment information technology with benefit potential (tangible preferred); total investment should be at or near levels of comparable hospitals.

I-5. Criteria: This strategy defines the hospital's criteria for evaluating and approving IT initiatives.
- Evaluate and approve IT initiatives based on sound cost or benefit criteria; both tangible and intangible benefits should be considered and should materially offset costs, but cost justification should not be dependent solely on tangible benefits.

■ II. Information System Acquisition and Implementation

II-1. Acquisition: This strategy defines the management team's preferred approach for obtaining new automated applications.
- For the most part, purchase vendor-supplied applications where feasible or acceptable; develop or contract for the development of the enhancements or customization of applications to fit the hospital's needs.

II-2. Customization: This strategy specifies the management team's preferred approach to tailoring or customizing applications to the hospital's specific needs.
- Systems should be highly responsive to user needs; customization done to fit the specific or unique needs.

II-3. Hardware: This strategy defines the management team's preferred approach to computer hardware selection.
- One primary computer manufacturer should be designated; hardware from other manufacturers is permitted but must be highly compatible with the technology standards set by the primary manufacturer, preference is given to applications running on the primary vendor's equipment.

II-4. Application Packaging: This strategy specifies the management team's preferred approach for grouping applications for evaluation and selection.
- Applications should be logically grouped for selection purposes whenever possible (such as general accounting, clinical support, patient management, and so forth); emphasis is on selecting by group but should be compatible with the primary source.

II-5. User Involvement: This strategy identifies the management team's willingness to commit operations personnel to system implementation projects.
- Key users are involved selectively; effort is concentrated in selection and procedural decision making; other project activities completed by IS staff.

II-6. Pacing: This strategy identifies the management team's preference for how quickly information system initiatives should occur to achieve defined benefits and support strategic goals.
- Move quickly in high priority areas; move slowly in others.

■ III. Technology Characteristics and Usage

III-1. Information Capture/Access: This strategy addresses the relative timeliness needed for information entry and retrieval.

Financial: Timely information capture and access are important, but use of on-line capabilities may be selective based on user needs, cost and benefits criteria; batched data entry or update is permitted where deemed appropriate; in some operating areas, reports and other printed output may serve as the primary means for information access.

Clinical: Timely information capture and access is very important; all systems should provide on-line entry and access to all required information; reports and other printed output should be available as needed to supplement on-line access.

III-2. Technology Currentness: This strategy specifies the degree to which the management team desires to keep current with technology advances in information processing.
- Periodically re-evaluate technology using cost and benefit guidelines.

■ IV. Systems Management and Support Services

IV-1. Executive Level Involvement: This strategy identifies the management team's willingness to actively participate in planning and managing information systems activities.

Executive level involvement provided through a steering committee that meets periodically and independently of other executive team meetings to address IT-related priorities, progress on projects and operational performance.

IV-2. Central Coordination: This strategy identifies the hospital's preference regarding the degree of central control to be exercised in managing information system planning, projects and ongoing operational support.

Central control focused on hospitalwide and/or interdepartmental IT activities; central coordination of department-specific initiatives to the extent needed to facilitate appropriate information sharing among systems.

IV-3. Customer Service: This strategy specifies the general guidelines for the scope of services or support to be provided by the IS Department.

User areas should be relatively self-sufficient; IS services or support should be principally focused on answering questions, addressing problems, operating centralized systems and assisting as needed with system implementation; major focus should be on technical support rather than functional or operational support.

V. Data Processing Action Plan Development

Priority Rating Factors	Rating
	5 = high priority; 1 = low priority
• High Benefit	4
• Low Cost	2
• High Visibility	3
• Low Risk of Failure	4
• Favorable Cost Benefit	3
• Political Sensitivity	1
• Support for Strategic Business Initiatives:	
- Expand the Number of Partner Providers	3

- Enhance Relationships with Current Medical Staff   3
- Improve Hospital Efficiency and Effectiveness   5
- Program Expansions (for example, Rehab, OB)   2

▪ Tentative Project List

- Access to Ferris/Internet
- Administrative LAN
    - Appointment calendars
    - E-Mail
    - Staff scheduling
    - WordPerfect®
- Advanced budgeting
- Application Integration Gateway (AIG)
- Cafeteria plan benefits administration
- Cashiering
- CD-ROM access to medical library information
- Centralized patient scheduling
- Chart tracking
- Clinical transcription
- Cost accounting
- Employee data processing training
    - Application specific
    - General (Lotus®, and so forth)
- Fetal monitor storage
- Full pharmacy system implementation and/or replacement
- Hospitalwide bar coding
- Housewide access to patient demographics and ADT
- Internal faxing of physician reports
- Laboratory system expansion or replacement
- Materials management (with satellite locations)
- Medical records imaging
- Medical staff credentialing
- Nutritional evaluation of menus
- On-line cash posting (back office)

- Order entry and results reporting
- Patient accounting optical storage upgrade
- Patient acuity system
- Patient care plans
- Physician access
- Radiology hardware expansion
- Report writer and data download capability
- Telephone logs (ER and OB)
- Therapist ID for productivity reporting (PT)
- Time and attendance (with cafeteria charging)

Departments Interviewed for Information-Management Plan

- Administration
- Administrative Secretary
- Quality Improvement
- Medical Staff Secretary
- Health Information Service
- Marketing
- Nursing
- Laboratory
- Radiology
- Cardiopulmonary
- Nutritional Services
- Pharmacy
- Accounting
- Patient Accounts
- Registration
- Specialty Clinics
- Material Services
- Environmental Services
- Bio-Medical
- Data Processing
- Education and Risk Management
- Board and Physicians

DATA PROCESSING PLAN OVERVIEW

The following calendar (see Figure 15, page 320) presents data processing in the order prioritized by the Project Team.

To prioritize the various projects, rating factors were established (such as cost, benefit, visibility, support for MCGH strategic business initiatives), and all projects were scored in each category and numerical values totalled. The resulting order of projects was used in conjunction with project dependencies (such as on-line order entry must be accomplished prior to point-of-service cashiering) to establish the overall project calendar.

The following is an estimate of the project-related costs by fiscal year as well as ongoing regular data processing capital requirements:

	Project-related	Ongoing
1995	$ 79,500	$30,000
1996	180,000	20,000
1997	90,600	15,000
1998	155,000	20,000
1999	95,000	15,000

It is important to note that the recommended project phases include numerous management and Board-level checkpoints to ensure that the projects remain on target and are responsive to the hospital's needs.

The following pages provide a brief description of each approved project in the plan with brief descriptions of those projects that were not approved or deferred at this time.

DATA PROCESSING PROJECT CALENDAR

The project calendar (see Figure 15) is a three to five year plan to be reviewed and or revised within that time.

Each department has been interviewed and all the projects were defined and an estimated dollar amount assigned. The administrative team defined the rating factors and prioritized the projects with the understanding certain projects had to be done before others.

The following is a list of the projects, estimated costs, and time frame to be completed.

ADT: Hooking up nursing to the AS/400 to be able to discharge and transfer patients from the floor eliminating the paperwork and hours to distribute the forms. The hardware would have been purchased by July 1994, and installed by August. Training should have been completed by October 1994 at the cost of $10,500.

Patient Accounts Optical Upgrade: The upgrade for the optical server to accommodate the archiving of patient bills and accounts receivable statuses. This is to maintain the efficiency of the department as it stands. The hardware would have been ordered in July 1994 and installed by October 1994 at the estimated cost of $15,000.

Pharmacy System Upgrade: The upgrade of the pharmacy package to have drug administration records, drug-to-drug interaction, and have drug education on the nursing floors. The planning for this project should have started in July 1994 and have been implemented by December 1994 at the cost of $4,000.

Administrative LAN: Purchasing a file server and linking PCs to it to share resources and communicate hospitalwide for such functions as word processing, calendars, and staff scheduling. The suggested word processor being WordPerfect. The estimated time for this project is six months, to begin in September 1994 at the cost of $35,000.

Chart Tracking: Additional functions for tracking physical location of patient charts and completion of all necessary entries into chart. This project should have started in August 1994 and

FIGURE 15 Mecosta County General Hospital Data Processing Project Calendar

Project	FY 1995				FY 1996				FY 1997				FY 1998				FY 1999			
	1	2	3	4	1	2	3	4	1	2	3	4	1	2	3	4	1	2	3	4
ADT/Patient Info Access			3																	
Pat. Acct Optical Upgrade		2	3																	
Pharmacy System Upgrade	1	2	3																	
Administrative LAN		1	2	3																
Chart Tracking		1	3																	
Order Entry/Result Rptg			1	2			3													
Physician Credentialing				1	2	3														
Clinical Transcription					1	2	3													
Centralized Scheduling						2	3													
Lab System Expansion									1	2	3									
Physician Access										2	3									
On-Line Cash Posting																				

Project Phases
1. Feasibility/requirements/selection
2. Implementation planning
3. Implementation

Appendix E Sample Information Management Plan **321**

FIGURE 15 Mecosta County General Hospital
Data Processing Project Calendar *(continued)*

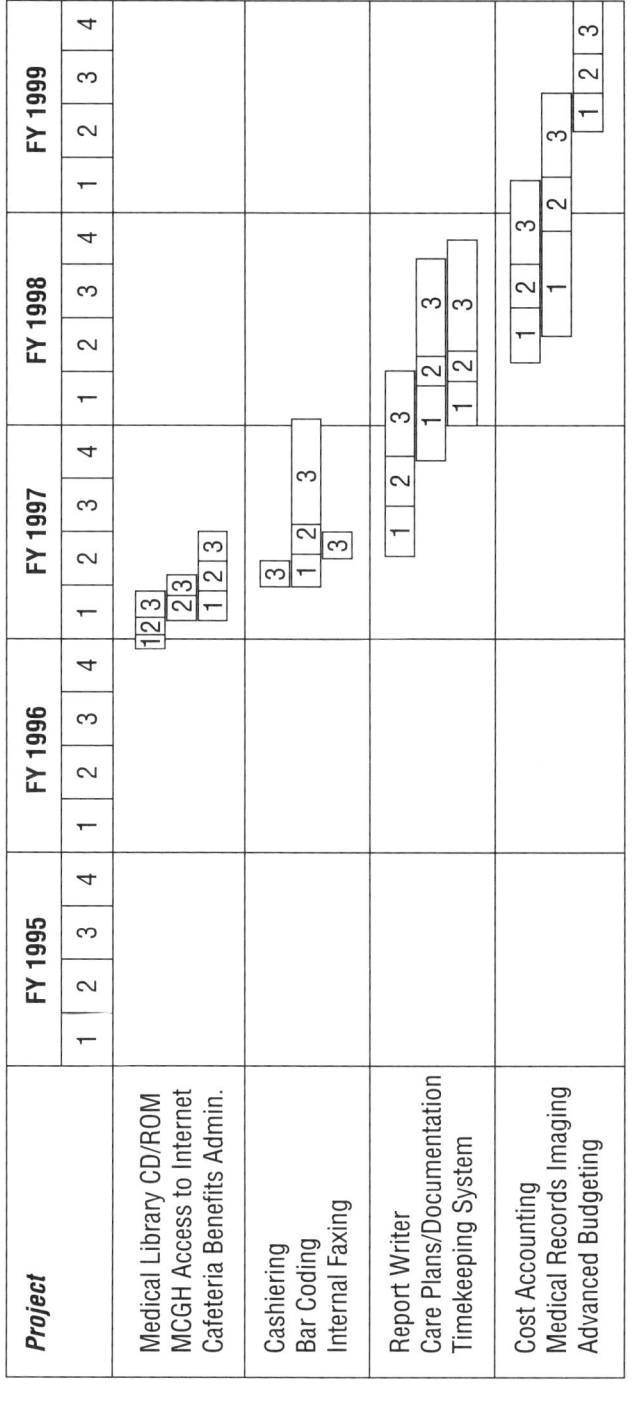

should have been completed by the end of September 1994 at the estimated cost of $3,000.

Order/Entry/Result Reporting: An application to allow the entry of patient orders from the nursing floor and communicate to the various departments to get the results back without nursing staff leaving the floor. The estimated time for this is 18 months to begin January 1995 at the estimated cost of $80,000.

Physician Credentialing: An application to administer the credentialing of physicians (for example, licensure and CME credits). This could reside on the administrative LAN. The estimated time of completion is four months beginning February 1995 at the cost of $5,000.

Clinical Transcription: The ability to transcribe all clinical data on the same software as that for everything else for the patient record. The estimated time is eight months to begin in June 1995 at the cost of $15,000.

Centralized Scheduling: The scheduling of patients done in a centralized area and shared with all departments. The estimated time is eight months to start August 1995 with the cost ranging from $25,000 to $40,000.

Lab System Expansion: The upgrade of the lab computer to accommodate the interface for order entry and result reporting. The estimated time is four months beginning in October 1995 at the cost of $45,000.

Physician Access: This access of patient demographics, ADT, and order entry and result reporting information for authorized physicians. The estimated time is 12 months beginning March 1996 at the cost of $3,000 per site. Estimating that total cost is up to $30,000.

On-Line Cash Posting: The posting of cash as the account is researched when the mail is received. The estimated time is two months starting July 1996 at the cost of $2,000.

Medical Library CD/ROM: The capability of the Medical Library search functions on CD/ROM within the hospital. The estimated time is three months starting December 1996 with the initial cost of $8,500 and a yearly fee of $5,000.

MCGH Access to Internet: A physical connection (via modem) to access the Internet of libraries through Ferris. The estimated cost is $2,500 and should take two months to complete starting August 1996.

Cafeteria Benefits Plan Administration: The ability to administer the personnel benefits (for example, child care, health care dollar bank) in house. The estimated time is five months beginning August 1996 at a cost of $2,000.

Cashiering: Posting cash and producing a bill at the time of service for all outpatient services. Collecting deductibles and personal pay amounts thereby reducing billing expense. The estimated time is one month beginning October 1996 at no additional cost.

Bar Coding: Implement bar coding hospitalwide to improve accuracy of patient identification and charges. The estimated time involved is ten months beginning October 1996 at a cost of up to $30,000.

Internal Faxing: Placing fax modems in PCs throughout the hospital to fax reports to physicians and businesses as deemed necessary. The estimated time involved is one month starting November 1996 at a cost of $150 each.

Report Writer: The ability to produce special reports on an individual basis upon demand. This project should take up to 12 months at a cost up to $15,000.

Care Plan and Documentation: The ability to set up care plans, implement them for each patient, and run reports for the acuity system. This project should take approximately 16 months starting March 1997 at a cost up to $60,000.

Timekeeping System: The ability to track employees from department to department and take cafeteria and pharmacy charges electronically and interface with the current payroll system. The estimated time and cost is 10 months starting July 1997 at a cost up to $25,000.

Cost Accounting: The ability to identify and report costs of each procedure, department, and DRG. This project should take 11 months starting October 1997 and cost $70,000.

Medical Records Imaging: The ability to store all the patients' medical records on optical storage in image format. This project should take 15 months beginning October 1998 at a cost up to $64,000.

Advanced Budgeting: The functions and features to facilitate the development and manipulation of various budgets, fixed and flexible. This project should take seven months beginning December 1998 at a cost of $30,000.

Application Integration Gateway: Hardware and software to facilitate the communications between different hardware and software application platforms. This project is out of our five-year plan and will be addressed in the future. The approximate cost is $100,000.

Employee Training by Data Processing: Training of all employees by Data Processing. At this time the Data Processing Department will train key people in each department and those people will be responsible of training all other employees.

Fetal Monitor Storage: This project will be addressed in the medical records imaging project.

Material Management: Inventory package to communicate with the rest of our financial package. The present package keeps inventory and produces purchase orders. The software has been written in a language that is difficult for us to communicate with. Servicemaster is working on a software package to fit on our network at this time.

Nutritional Evaluation of Menus: Evaluation of menus from a nutritional standpoint. This project is department specific and felt that the software is probably provided from the purchased service elsewhere. We recommend that Hospital Dietary Service check with their programmers.

Telephone Logs: Log phone conversations for follow up at a later date. This project was too department specific to use a general program. It is suggested the conversations be kept on a PC in the department as to the specific information requested.

Therapist ID for Productivity: Assigning ID numbers to the physical therapists to track productivity. This project is department specific and should be addressed when doing documentation in the package provided from the purchased service.

Index

A
Access control mechanisms, 42
Aggregate data and information (IM.8), 90–99, 247–265
Ambulatory care visits (IM.7.10), 88–90, 243–246
Ambulatory patients (IM.7.5), 82–83
Appointment system (IM.8.1.6.1), 95–96, 249–250, 259–260
Audit log, 42
Authoritative resources, 106

B
Backup and recovery mechanisms, 42

C
Clinical research (IM.8.1.12), 98–99, 250, 265
Coding systems, 47, 95–96, 186–189, 248, 249–250, 257–258, 260–261
Comparative data and information (IM.10), 111–114, 276–281
Cycle for Improving Performance, 117

D
Data and information. *See* Management of information, standards on
Data collection
  methods (IM.3), 46–53, 186–196
  timeliness, accuracy, and efficiency of (IM.3.2), 46–53, 186–190
Data dictionary, 50–51
Data inventory, 49
Dial-back modems, 42
Dimensions of Performance, 37, 118–119
Disaster recovery plan, 45–46
Discharge, clinical resume for (IM.7.3), 77–79, 213–215
Discretionary access control, 42

E
Emergency care (IM.7.6), 83–84
  control register for (IM.8.1.6.1), 95–96, 249–250, 259–260
  emergency care visits (IM.7.10), 88–90, 243–246
Encryption, 42
External environment, 19–21

F
Framework for Improving Performance, 18–22

327

H

Health care networks, 1–2, 27–28
Healthy People 2000 Report, 174

I

IMSystem (Indicator Measurement System), 113, 283–287
  confidentiality, 287
  participation, 286–287
  technology requirements, 284–285
  use of data, 285–286
Information management. *See also* Management of information, standards on
  flowchart for, 12, 165
  processes for, 3–4, 11, 171–175
  processes versus technology, 13–15
  rationale and theory of, 1–3, 171–173
  sample plan, 311–325
Institute of Medicine, 174
Internal environment, 19–21
Invasive procedures (IM.7.4), 80–82, 216–224

J

Joint Commission
  Board of Commissioners, 9
  contacting, 5

K

Knowledge-based information (IM.9), 100–111, 265–276

L

Library, 104, 106

M

Management of information, standards on, 23–121, 171–281. *See also* Information management
  access to external databases (IM.6.3), 67–71, 201–206
  aggregate data and information (IM.8), 90–99, 247–265
  appointment system for outpatient services (IM.8.1.6.1), 95–96, 249–250, 259–260
  coding and retrieval systems (IM.8.1.5), 95–96, 248, 250–251, 257–258
  control register for emergency services (IM.8.1.6.1), 95–96, 249–250, 259–260
  external regulatory requirements (IM.8.1.4), 94–95, 248, 250–251, 256–257
  financial information coding and retrieval (IM.8.1.7), 95–96, 249–250, 260–261
  hazards and unsafe practices (IM.8.1.2.2), 93, 248, 250, 253–255
  independent practitioner-specific data (IM.8.1.10), 97–98, 249–250, 263–264
  medical records coding and retrieval (IM.8.1.5), 95–96, 248, 250, 257–258
  occupational illness (IM.8.1.2.3), 93–94, 248, 250, 255
  operational decision making and planning, for (IM.8.1.11), 98–99, 249–250, 264

patient demographic information (IM.8.1.6), 95–96, 248–250, 258–260
patient, personnel, or visitor injury (IM.8.1.2.3), 93–94, 248, 250, 255
performance improvement activities summaries (IM.8.1.9), 96–97, 249–250, 262–263
pharmacy transactions (IM.8.1.1), 92–94, 247, 250, 252
practitioner credentialing (IM.8.1.10), 97–98, 249, 250–251, 263–264
practitioners' DEA numbers (IM.8.1.1.2), 92–94, 247, 250, 252
process and outcome measures for assessing performance (IM.8.1.8), 96–97, 249–250, 261–262
property damage (IM.8.1.2.3), 93, 248, 250, 255
radionuclide disposal (IM.8.1.3), 94, 248, 250, 256
radiopharmaceutical disposal (IM.8.1.3), 94, 248, 250, 256
required reporting to proper authorities (IM.8.1.4), 94–95, 248, 250, 256–257
requirements for (IM.8.1), 91–92, 247–265
safety information (IM.8.1.2.1), 93–94, 248, 250, 253
signature identification, for medication orders (IM.8.1.1.1), 92–94, 247, 250, 252
support clinical research, to (IM.8.1.12), 98–99, 250, 265

survey for, 92
appropriateness of processes (IM.1.1), 24, 177–179
codes, classifications, and terminology (IM.3.1), 46–53, 186–189
comparative data and information (IM.10), 111–114, 276–281
application example, 118–121
external reference databases (IM.10.1), (IM.10.2), 111–114, 276–280
performance measures grid, 120
quality cube, 119
security and confidentiality (IM.10.3), 111–114, 276–281
sources of, 277–279
survey for, 113
data and information
accuracy assessment (IM.3.3), 46–53, 186–191
bias minimization in (IM.3.3), 46–53, 186–191
confidentiality (IM.2), 38–46, 180–185
requirements for, 39
survey for, 39–40
data security features, 42
integration, linkage (IM.6), 67–71, 200–206
requirements for, 68–69
survey for, 69
integrity (IM.2), 38–46, 180–185
methods for capturing (IM.3), 46–53, 186–196
requirements for, 47–48
survey for, 48–52
reliability assessment (IM.3.3), 46–53, 186–191
safeguarding (IM.2), 38–46, 180–185

security (IM.2), 38–46,
    180–185
transmission, timeliness, and
    accuracy (IM.5), 63–66,
    198–200
  requirements for, 63–64
  survey for, 64–65
  validity assessment (IM.3.3),
    46–53, 186–191
data collection
  methods (IM.3), 46–53,
    186–196
  timeliness, accuracy, and
    efficiency of (IM.3.2),
    46–53, 186–190
direction (IM.1.1.1), 177–179
education and training of
    responsible individuals
    (IM.4), 58–63, 196–198
  application example, 62
  requirements for, 58–59
  survey for, 59
knowledge-based information
    (IM.9), 100–111, 265–276
  accessibility (IM.9.2),
    (IM.9.4), 102–105, 268–271,
    273–275
  hospital formulary or drug
    list information (IM.9.6),
    103–105, 275
  linkage with external
    databases and information
    networks (IM.9.2),
    102–103, 268–271
  linkage with internal
    information systems
    (IM.9.2), 102–103, 268–271
  needs-related (IM.9.2),
    102–103, 268–271
  organization of (IM.9.1),
    102–103, 266–268
  planning for (IM.9.1),
    102–103, 268–271
  poison-control information
    (IM.9.5), 103–105, 275
  requirements for (IM.9),
    100–101
  resources (IM.9.4), 103–105,
    273–275
  sample survey for, 107–111
  survey for, 101
  systems and structures
    (IM.9.3), 103–105, 271–273
  timeliness (IM.9.2.1.1),
    102–103, 268–271
knowledge-based resources
    (IM.6.3), 67–71, 201–206
linkages in (IM.6), 67–71,
    200–206
medical record review
    (IM.3.3.1), 54–58, 191–196
medical records (IM.7.1),
    (IM.7.2), 74–77, 207,
    209–212
  authentication of entries
    (IM.7.9), 87–88, 239–243
  timely completion of record
    (IM.7.7), 84–85, 229–234
patient-specific data and
    information (IM.7), 72–90,
    206–246
  ambulatory care visits
    (IM.7.10), 88–90, 243–246
  ambulatory patients (IM.7.5),
    82–83, 224–226
  assembly of divergently
    located components
    (IM.7.10), 88–90, 243–246
  clinical resume at discharge
    (IM.7.3), 77–79, 213–215
  discharge information
    (IM.7.3), 77, 213–215
  emergency care (IM.7.6),
    83–84
  emergency care visits
    (IM.7.10), 88–90, 243–246
  medical record. *See* Medical
    records
  operative or other invasive
    procedures (IM.7.4), 80,
    215–224

postoperative, requirements
for (IM.7.4.3), 80–82,
216–224
requirements for, 72–73
retrieval (IM.7.10), 88–90,
243–246
survey for, 73
transfer summary (IM.7.3.2),
77–79, 213–215
verbal orders (IM.7.8), 86–87,
235–239
performance improvement
(PI.3.4), 114–121
survey for, 115–116
planning for, 23–37, 175–206
application example, 31–37
assessment of needs (IM.1),
23–24, 175–177
checklist for, 27
material resource allocation
for (IM.1.1.1), 24, 177–179
requirements for, 24–25
staff involvement, 29–30
survey for, 25–31
technology assessment,
selection, and
integration (IM.1.1.2), 24,
177–180
processes for, 171–175
rationale and theory of,
171–173
staff (IM.1.1.1), 177–179
standardized minimum data
sets (IM.3.1), 46–53,
186–189
survey probes for, 132–136
uniform data definitions
(IM.3), 46–53, 186–196
Mandatory access control, 42
Medical records (IM.7.1),
(IM.7.2), 74–77
authentication of entries
(IM.7.9), 87–88, 239–242
coding and retrieval (IM.8.1.5),
95–96, 248, 250, 257–258
divergent record components
(IM.7.10), 88–90
required information for, 78
review of (IM.3.3.1), 54–58,
191–196
checklist for, 55
requirements for, 54–56
survey for, 56
timely completion (IM.7.7),
84–85
Minimum data sets (IM.3.1), 47,
186–189
Multidisciplinary review, 56

O

Occupational illness (IM.8.1.2.3),
248, 250, 255
Operative procedures
(IM.7.2.13), 80–82, 208–216
Organizational function, 11–13
Outpatient services,
appointment system for
(IM.8.1.6.1), 95–96,
249–250, 259–260

P

Passwords, 42
Patient-specific data and
information (IM.7), 72–90,
206–246
Performance assessment and
improvement (PL.3.4), 8,
15–17, 114–121
activities summaries (IM.8.1.9),
96–97, 249–250, 262–263
application example, 118–121
cycle for, 21–22, 116–117
framework for, 18–22
indicators for, 117–118
process and outcome measures
(IM.8.1.8), 96–97, 249–250,
261–262
quality cube, 119

survey for, 115–118
Pharmacy transactions (IM.8.1.1), 92–94, 247, 250, 252
Poison-control information (IM.9.5), 103–105, 275
Postoperative care (IM.7.4.3), 80–82, 216–224
Processes versus technology, 13–15
Property damage (IM.8.1.2.3), 248, 250, 255

R

Radionuclide disposal (IM.8.1.3), 248, 250, 256
Radiopharmaceutical disposal (IM.8.1.3), 248, 250, 256
Request for proposal (RFP), 30–31

S

Scoring scale, 16
Security features, 42
  examples of, 42
Security guards, gateways, intelligent routers, 42
Software Specifications manual, 284–285
Staff (IM.1.1.1), 23–24, 177–179
  education and training (IM.4), 58–63, 196–198
Standards
  development of, 7–10
  emphasis on performance, 15–17
  future changes, 17–18
  meeting information needs, 10–11
  organizational function, 11–13
  overview, 7–22
  planning guide, as, 10
  scoring, 16
Survey probes, 132–136
Survey process, 123–161
  applicable standards by department/service, 145
  building tour, 144
  closed medical record form, 147–150
  consistency of, 124
  document review, 136–137
  documents typically requested, 138–139
  emphasis on education, 126
  feedback activities, 160
  inpatient unit visits, 140–142
  interactive process, 125–126
  interviews, 137, 142–144, 146–160
  introductory sessions, 136
  leadership interview, 137
  length of, 126
  management of information interview, 142–143
  medical record interview, 146–160
  other care area visits, 142
  other interviews, 144
  patient care settings visit, 139–142
  post-survey activities, 161
  pre-survey activities, 126–127
  resource center visit, 160
  sample agenda for survey, 128–131
  step-by-step through survey, 126–161
  survey probes, 132–136
  tailoring of, 124
  tally for closed medical record forms, 151–159
  team-based approach, 125

T

Technology
  data security features, 42
  IMSystem requirements, 284–285
  processes versus, 13–15
Training, 58–63, 196–198
Transaction log, 42

U

Uniform data definitions, 47, 52–53, 66, 186–196
User identification and authentication, 42

V

Verbal orders (IM.7.8), 86–87, 235–239